The East in the Light of the West

Two Eastern Streams of the Twentieth Century in the Light of Christian Esotericism

Part 1: Agni Yoga

Sergei O. Prokofieff

TEMPLE LODGE
London

Translated from the Russian by Simon Blaxland de Lange

Temple Lodge Publishing
51 Queen Caroline Street
London W6 9QL

First English edition 1993

Originally published in German under the title *Der Osten im Lichte des Westens, Zwei östliche Strömungen im 20. Jahrhundert aus der Sicht der Christlichen Esoterik, Teil 1* by Philosophisch-Anthroposophischer Verlag am Goetheanum, Dornach in 1992

A catalogue record for this book is available from the British Library

ISBN 0 904693 57 0

Cover by S. Gulbekian. Photograph of Nicholas Roerich and his son George Roerich in Tibetan costume reproduced by permission of Hulton Deutsch

Typeset by DP Photosetting, Aylesbury, Bucks

Printed and bound in Great Britain by Cromwell Press Limited, Broughton Gifford, Wiltshire

Contents

Preface

In the year that these words are being written (1991), the hundredth anniversary of the death of H.P. Blavatsky (1831–91), the founder of the Theosophical Society, is being marked in the many countries of the world where this Society exists. Especially in the last years of her life, Blavatsky frequently alluded to the Indo-Tibetan occult teachers – whom she called the Mahatmas – who stood behind her and instructed her. Two in particular of these have been highly revered in the Theosophical Society. In the first half of the 20th century, frequent attempts were made to enter again into direct contact with them. In certain cases these efforts were apparently successful, and as a result new occult streams inspired by them have arisen which continue to stimulate interest – and also interest in Blavatsky herself and in her works – to this day. Two of these streams will be considered in the present study from an anthroposophical point of view. These are the occult stream of Agni Yoga, founded by the Russian, Helena Roerich, and that other occult stream founded on the teachings of the Englishwoman Alice Bailey, which have also been largely responsible for inspiring the essential philosophy of the so-called 'New Age' movement.

In the present publication, only the first of these streams will be considered. A study of the second will follow in the second part, which will be published separately.

Introduction

Amongst all the many occult streams which have in recent years become widespread and even officially acknowledged in Russia, the spiritual movement originating in Helena and Nicholas Roerich occupies a particular place.

There are at present in Russia, Latvia and Byelorussia several officially registered Roerich societies: in Moscow, Petrozavodsk, Novosibirsk, Riga, Minsk, St Petersburg and so on. Active publishing and propaganda work is being pursued. Books and journals are being published, symposiums and exhibitions are being organised – in brief, the cultural, artistic and occult legacy of the Roerichs is being disseminated and popularised in every possible way.

The Gorbachevs also appear to have a certain interest in the legacy of the Roerichs. They have met Nicholas Roerich's son, Svyatoslav (who until his recent death was living in India) in both India and Moscow, and have visited the Roerich Museum in New York. The two meetings in Moscow with the artist's son – which took place in the Kremlin in May 1987 and October 1989 – were of particular significance. 'This meeting has long been a wish of ours', said Gorbachev at the first of them;[1] and during the second he declared: 'In the Soviet Union the memory of Nicholas Roerich is cherished with deep gratitude . . .'[2] In a brochure advertising the publication of the German translation of the large monograph on the life and work of Nicholas Roerich recently published in America, the following words are quoted which Gorbachev spoke about the Russian artist in November 1989, that is, immediately after the second meeting with his son: 'Nicholas Roerich was a man who brought glory to our people; he is a representative of our civilisation and of its culture, one of its pillars.'[3]* Moreover, the publication of this book testifies to the ever growing interest in the legacy of Roerich in both Switzerland and Germany. In the latter country there has been a society named after him for the last few years; and on its initiative all the books and two volumes of Helena Roerich's letters have been translated into German. The centre of the movement in America is the Roerich Museum in New York. Almost all the writings of Helena and Nicholas Roerich have long been available in English, and many of their books have also been translated into other European and even Eastern languages.

The principal purpose of what follows is not so much to consider the outer biography of the Roerichs as to attempt to reveal the sources of the occult stream which is associated with their name.

---

* See Supplement 1.

1. The Sources of the Later Teachings of H.P. Blavatsky

The occult stream initiated at the beginning of the 1920s by Helena Roerich (1879–1951), the wife of the artist Nicholas Roerich (1874–1947), was called by her 'Agni Yoga' or the 'Teaching of Living Ethics'. She expounded it in fourteen volumes, thirteen of which were published in Russian in Paris and Riga between 1924 and 1938, while the fourteenth for a long time existed only in manuscript form and was only recently published for the first time in Russian. The two collected volumes of letters (1929–38) of Helena Roerich to her spiritual pupils and followers, which are a kind of commentary to it, were also brought out in Russian in Riga in the year 1940. In these letters she replies at some length to various questions relating to one or another aspect of the teaching. It is evident from the letters that in the thirties there were groups studying the teaching of Agni Yoga in many countries in Europe and America. The Roerichs started establishing these groups in 1920.[4]

At the present time, similar groups are active in many of the towns of Russia and of other republics. The volumes of *Agni Yoga* are appearing simultaneously in Riga, Moscow, St Petersburg, Novosibirsk, Tbilisi and Samara; while the journal of the Latvian Roerich Society, *Uguns*, which is brought out in Riga in Russian and Latvian, tells of the many activities undertaken by the Society and also of the work with children and adolescents on mastering the essentials of the teaching that it carries out.

The very name of the teaching – 'Agni Yoga' or 'yoga of fire' – testifies to its Eastern origin. However, the Roerichs did not find their way to it at once but only gradually, through their well-known compatriot, Helena Petrovna Blavatsky, the founder of the Theosophical Society. The first lodge of this society was opened in Russia in 1908. And, as the American, Jacqueline Decter, writes in her monograph on Nicholas Roerich, 'the Roerichs apparently joined it [the Russian branch of the Theosophical Society] prior to World War I.'[5]

As a result of becoming acquainted with theosophical literature and above all with the writings of Blavatsky herself, the Roerichs first came in contact with the ultimate source of her inspiration, which can be traced back to mysterious mahatmas or teachers of the East who lived somewhere in one of the remote villages of the central Himalayas but who from time to time ventured to Europe and America.

According to Blavatsky, two in particular of these mahatmas spiritually guided her and inspired the writing of her main and most extensive work, *The Secret Doctrine*. Helena Roerich subsequently translated it into Russian and published the first two volumes in Riga under the imprint of the same publishing house which brought out the books relating to Agni Yoga.

Since Helena Roerich herself often pointed out that the inspirations which she received were derived from the same source as those of Blavatsky, it is necessary to attempt briefly to characterise this source from an anthroposophical point of view on the basis of Rudolf Steiner's spiritual-scientific research. Thus Rudolf Steiner characterised the inner nature of the Theosophical Society – which had been founded in New York in 1875 – in a letter to the French writer and theosophist, Edouard Schuré.* It is clear from this manuscript

---

* See Supplement VII.

that Helena Blavatsky had originally been inspired by 'the great initiates of the West, who were also the initiators of Rosicrucian wisdom'. Her first substantial book, *Isis Unveiled*, was written out of this source of inspiration; and the Theosophical Society, which initially had as its chief purpose the service of the highest ideals of humanity, was also founded in the spirit of Rosicrucianism.[6]

However, because of her chaotic character, her lack of logical thinking and her inadequate control over her own considerable mediumistic faculties, Helena Blavatsky was only able, in the book referred to above, to give expression to Rosicrucian wisdom in a very incomplete, and in many respects even distorted, form. That her conscious insight into this wisdom remained at a not very elevated level is, for example, evident from the fact that in *Isis Unveiled* there is no mention of reincarnation; for this truth was in the Rosicrucian Mysteries accessible only at higher stages of inner development,[7] and these were beyond Blavatsky's reach.

When, shortly after the founding of the Theosophical Society, it became clear that high spiritual truths could only be communicated by Blavatsky in a distorted form, the Rosicrucian initiates ceased to inspire her and soon broke off all contact with her.

Nevertheless, Blavatsky's faculty for receiving higher inspirations – albeit in a mediumistic way – did not forsake her. The gates of her soul were now wide open and 'Eastern initiators were able to take hold of her'. 'Under the influence of this stream, the Theosophical Society took on its Eastern character, and Sinnett's *Esoteric Buddhism* and Blavatsky's *Secret Doctrine* were inspired by this same influence.'[8]

There were at least three reasons why, despite Blavatsky's estrangement from the sources of the Christian esotericism which belongs to all mankind, Rudolf Steiner was – especially in his early lectures – able to speak positively about the founder of the Theosophical Society. For in the first place, 'this initial foundation had a clearly defined Western [i.e. Rosicrucian] character';[9] in the second place, because much that Blavatsky imparted also in her later writings stemmed from her own occult experiences (for although her supersensible faculties were of a mediumistic character, she was nevertheless able to perceive certain spiritual realities); and, in the third place, because much of what is imparted in *The Secret Doctrine* regarding pre-Christian religions and the former conditions of the Earth and humanity had objective philosophical value. Finally, considerable personal courage must have been necessary on Blavatsky's part to dare to speak publicly on occult themes at all in the second half of the 19th century, in the period when Euro-American materialism had reached its culmination, even if what she said was couched in a non-Christian form.

However, when 'the ice was broken' from the Eastern side, Western Christian occultism was able to speak forth through Rudolf Steiner with full force. He speaks of this as follows: 'Once the ice was broken in the way that I have indicated [through the publication of Blavatsky's *The Secret Doctrine*], the time had also come when it was possible to speak ... out of the sources of living occultism, which has been faithfully guarded in the Rosicrucian mysteries.'[10] And then in the same lecture, Rudolf Steiner speaks about the main difference between Western and Eastern occultism: 'There is no such thing as an Eastern wisdom which is unknown to Western occultism, and in Rosicrucian teaching and research you will find to the last jot everything that has at one time or another been assimilated by the great sages of the East. Nothing of what it is possible to know from Eastern wisdom is lacking in the wisdom of the West ... It is simply that it [Western occultism] *had to renew all things through the rejuvenating spring of the Christ-impulse.*'

It follows from this that Blavatsky's succumbing to the influence of Eastern occultism with their Indo-Tibetan group interests necessarily led to a whole series of highly negative consequences, the occult significance and spiritual basis of which Rudolf Steiner was able to reveal to anthroposophists only much later, after the break with the Theosophical Society.

In the lectures which he gave at Dornach in October 1915, published under the title *The Occult Movement in the Nineteenth Century*,* Rudolf Steiner described at greater length the whole process of Blavatsky's coming under the influence of Eastern initiates. Here he related how, as a result of Blavatsky's membership of various occult brotherhoods of Europe and America (which often tried to make use of her for the attainment of their group egotistical and even political aims) and also because of her – essentially honest but – very emotional and unbalanced character, she eventually became altogether ungovernable by, and therefore highly dangerous to, the brotherhoods into whose many secrets she had been initiated. Because of the thoroughly confused and critical situation that had arisen, certain Western brotherhoods resolved upon the drastic remedy of subjecting Blavatsky to what in esoteric circles is called 'occult imprisonment'. This essentially consists of the following. With the help of certain devices of ceremonial magic, the soul of the person concerned is surrounded on the astral plane by a supersensible sheath or aura which reflects back all the impulses which the imprisoned soul wishes to send into the world. In other words, Blavatsky

---

* GA 254.

was inwardly placed in such a position that all her vast occult knowledge was thrust back into her soul by the spiritual sheath that had been formed around her. She was then rescued from this difficult situation by Eastern Indo-Tibetan occultists, by so-called mahatmas whose activity was, however, guided by specific group-egotistical interests rather than by those of a universally human dimension.* Henceforth Blavatsky became an obedient instrument in their hands, and subsequently the principal mediator between these Indo-Tibetan mahatmas and the leading members of the Theosophical Society: A.P. Sinnett, Colonel Olcott, C.W. Leadbeater, Annie Besant and others. This came symbolically to expression in that in 1879 the centre of the Theosophical Society was transferred from New York to India, to Madras, where Blavatsky herself now moved (she remained in India until 1886).†

From the inspirations of these mahatmas and with their help were subsequently written Sinnett's *The Occult World*, which also contained a number of the mahatmas' letters to the author (1881); his *Esoteric Buddhism* (1883); and Blavatsky's *The Secret Doctrine* (1888). The chief quality of the latter two – the most authoritative books in theosophical circles – was their distinctive mixture of 'Indian esotericism' and 'modern materialistic science', a mixture which Rudolf Steiner, in the notes that he made for Schuré, called 'a barren hybrid'.[11] As a result of this both works acquired a strongly materialistic timbre. Thus Rudolf Steiner says of Sinnett's *Esoteric Buddhism* that 'efforts were being made from a certain quarter to give an entirely materialistic form to [Eastern] spiritual teaching ... [In this book one finds] materialism in one of its very worst forms.

* See Supplement II.

† See Supplement III.

The spiritual world is presented here in an entirely materialistic way ... The subject-matter is, of course, very refined, but in Sinnett's book one cannot get away from materialism, however lofty the heights to which one may be led.'[12] Rudolf Steiner then goes on to speak about Blavatsky's principal work as follows: 'This [book], *The Secret Doctrine*, is written in the same style as *Esoteric Buddhism*'. And somewhat earlier in the same lecture he characterises Blavatsky's situation in the following words: 'And so those who now were H.P. B[lavatsky]'s spiritual "proprietors" – forgive the materialistic analogy – not only had special aims connected with Indian interests but also made trenchant concessions to the materialistic spirit of the age'.

In one respect, however, Blavatsky's book was at variance with that of Sinnett – namely, in its view of the Moon's significance in connection with the so-called 'eighth sphere' or the sphere of evil. Thus on the basis of information that he had apparently received from one of the mahatmas, Sinnett asserted in his book that the physical Moon itself is the eighth sphere. Actually, the contrary is true. The physical Moon orbits the Earth precisely as a means of *countering* the evil forces of the eighth sphere. According to Rudolf Steiner, with this erroneous assertion of Sinnett 'materialism is introduced into the realm of occultism and occultism becomes materialism'.[13] 'And so it was easy for that individuality, whose interest lay in making use of materialism in a spiritual way for particular purposes of his own, to disseminate in Sinnett's *Esoteric Buddhism* an ostensibly spiritual teaching with a very strong materialistic hue.'[14] And in another lecture Rudolf Steiner continues this thought as follows: 'Someone – and in this case this is not Mr Sinnett but whoever stands behind him – who has an interest in moulding earthly life in such a way that materialism becomes super-materialism is responsible for bringing this [false] teaching about the Moon . . .'[15]

Blavatsky, however – in contrast to Sinnett, who did not have any spiritual experience of his own – possessed real clairvoyant faculties, albeit of a mediumistic kind, and therefore 'was well aware that what Sinnett had written was untrue'.[16] And as she was essentially a deeply honest person (as has been pointed out), she could not agree with this. 'But on the other hand she was in the hands of those who desired that the false teaching [about the Moon] should be inculcated into humanity.'[17] Nevertheless, even though she was 'in the hands of' the Indo-Tibetan occultists, she tried in her book *The Secret Doctrine* to rectify this error to some extent, although in such a way that as a result of this partial rectification 'not too much harm should be done to the stream of Indian occultism'.[18] Thus Blavatsky, as it were 'in exchange', agreed to yield to the Indian occultists in another, still more important respect, as a result of which 'Blavatsky corrected [Sinnett's error] in a way that sought to reinforce the one-sidedness of the left-wing Indian occultists'.[19] Having rectified (in her book) Sinnett's error by correctly pointing out that the Moon is not the eighth sphere but has, on the contrary, been placed in the cosmos by the Gods as a counterweight to the forces of evil proceeding from the eighth sphere, Blavatsky at the same time presented in the same book an altogether false teaching about Jahve, that is, about that mighty Being who – as the spiritual ruler of the Moon – is also the chief antagonist of the eighth sphere.

As she had – under the influence of her Indo-Tibetan inspirers – completely distorted the truth about Jahve, Blavatsky had actually ceased to be able to understand either Judaism or Christianity, despite the fact that in her first book, *Isis Unveiled*, she had already given expression to certain truths of esoteric Judaism and Christianity. The result of this was that 'in *The Secret Doctrine* she gave vent to a volley of abuse about everything to do with Judaism and Christianity.'[20]

Rudolf Steiner describes this process of Blavatsky's transformation into an implacable opponent of Judaism and Christianity in the following words: 'In order to establish on her own account something that would outweigh Sinnett's assertion [about the Moon], she [Blavatsky] acceded to the proposals of the Indian occultists who were inspiring her. These occultists, being adherents of the left path, had no other aim than the promotion of their own specifically Indian interests. They had in mind to establish over the entire Earth a system of wisdom from which Christ, and also Jahve or Jehovah, were excluded. And so something which would gradually eliminate Christ and Jahve had to be secretly interpolated in her teaching.'[21]

In order to understand how these intentions came to exist amongst the Eastern occultists, it is necessary to bear in mind that it was fundamentally impossible for the Eastern initiate to approach a true knowledge of the Christ Mysteries. Rudolf Steiner refers to this in the notes that he made for Schuré: 'For the Eastern initiations must necessarily leave the *Christ-principle*, the central *cosmic* factor in evolution, untouched'. Thus 'they ['the revelations of Eastern initiation' and the mahatmas who stand behind them] can only hope for success in evolution if they can eradicate the Christ-principle from Western culture. This would, however, be equivalent to nullifying the *meaning of the Earth*, which consists in the knowledge and the fulfilment of the intentions of the *living Christ*.'[22]*

As a means of achieving the purposes of the Indo-Tibetan initiates through Blavatsky, the attempt was made to replace the impulse of Christ-Jahve by the impulse of Lucifer: 'The

---

* In both quotations, the italics are Rudolf Steiner's. (See Supplement VII.)

following method was then adopted. It was said: If we consider Lucifer – nothing was said about Ahriman; so little was known about him that one name was used for both – we see what a great benefactor of mankind he is. He brings to men everything they have gained through the head: science, art, in short, all progress. He is the true spirit of light, and it is to him that we must adhere ... Hence, [Blavatsky's] assertion in *The Secret Doctrine* that men should not adhere to Jahve, for ... the true benefactor of mankind is Lucifer. The whole of *The Secret Doctrine* is built up in such a way that this notion shimmers through it and is also clearly expressed in it. And so for occult reasons Blavatsky had to be made into someone who hated Christ-Jahve. For in the occult domain this has exactly the same significance as the statement that the Moon is the eighth sphere has in the realm that Sinnett was concerned with.' In other words, 'what it was desired to achieve through Blavatsky was, similarly, to mislead people into believing in the eighth sphere'.[23]

Thus through turning Blavatsky into an opponent of Christianity, the Indo-Tibetan mahatmas managed to make the theosophical movement completely anti-Christian and avowedly *luciferic*. 'Of course, people were led in this way to the spiritual world; and this was *The Secret Doctrine*'s great merit ... But this path was such that it pursued only specific – as opposed to universally human – interests in the evolution of mankind.'[24]

Bearing in mind the considerable importance of this process, let us now consider a further description of it, this time from the lecture of 27 November 1916: 'Blavatsky was misled by certain beings whose aim it was to allure her into replacing Christ by Lucifer; this was to come about through spreading ideas about the eighth sphere which were the complete opposite of the truth and through maligning the God, Jahve, whom they made out to be a god of a lower order. Thus those cosmic powers that sought to further materialism were also working on behalf of materialism through what was called Theosophy, for materialism would have plunged to the most abysmal depths if people had believed that the Moon really is the eighth sphere . . . and that it is necessary to do battle with Christianity.'[25]

It follows from what Rudolf Steiner says here that from the time when the centre of the Theosophical Society was transferred to India, and especially after the appearance of the books of Sinnett and Blavatsky that have been referred to, strongly materialistic tendencies arose within the theosophical movement which in subsequent years were to be developed to an increasing degree. Their culmination was the whole affair connected with the Indian boy, Krishnamurti, whom Leadbeater and Besant tried from 1909 onwards to claim as the new messiah, as a reincarnation of Christ.

The source of this 'occult adventure' is to be found above all in the general materialistic and anti-Christian tendencies of the theosophical movement, and can ultimately be traced back to that strictly enclosed group of Indo-Tibetan mahatmas, two of whom – according to Blavatsky and Sinnett – were the direct inspirers of *The Secret Doctrine* and *Esoteric Buddhism*. In theosophical circles these mahatmas were known under the names of M. (Morya) and K.H. (Kut Humi). The former is said to have inspired the aforesaid book of Blavatsky, while the latter, through his correspondence with Sinnett, laid the foundation for his (Sinnett's) books. Portraits of both mahatmas – the higher patrons of the Theosophical Society – always hung at the premises of the esoteric school founded by Blavatsky in India in the year of *The Secret Doctrine*'s publication (1888).

2. The Inspirers of Agni Yoga

From the time when they first became acquainted with the theosophical movement and above all with the works of Blavatsky and Sinnett, it was the chief aim of the Roerichs to enter into direct connection with its Eastern inspirers. This contact was indeed soon established, and the founding of Agni Yoga was the result. In the present work we shall leave open the question as to *who* it was who inspired Helena Roerich to write the fourteen volumes of *Agni Yoga*. She was in any case utterly convinced that this was *Mahatma Morya*.* Nicholas Roerich fully shared this opinion, as is – to cite one example – clear from the title of the collection of poems which he published in Berlin in 1921 (and had written between 1916 and 1921), *Tsvyety Morii* ('Flowers of Morya').[26] The collection consists of four parts, in which man's path from the first steps of pupilship to becoming a teacher, or guru, is described in the form of a poetic allegory.

As for Helena Roerich, she records in the eighth volume of *Agni Yoga* the following answer of the mahatmas to the question as to the common source of her teaching and that of

---

* In the present work the author has not considered it his task to identify the personalities of the theosophical teachers bearing the names of Morya and Kut Humi. His aim has simply been to indicate the quite particular intentions which have proceeded from those individualities (whoever they may have been) whom H. Roerich (and also, as we shall see, A. Bailey) called by these names (following Blavatsky), and whom she regarded as her 'mahatmas'. In an esoteric sense they are the founders of those occult streams to the study of which the present work is devoted.

Blavatsky: 'It may be asked what is the relationship of Our Teaching to that [teaching] given to Us through Blavatsky? Shall we say that in every century there ensues, after a full exposition, a final culmination ... Thus Our Teaching includes [within itself] the *Secret Doctrine* of Blavatsky'.[27] By 'full exposition' here is evidently meant Blavatsky's book, and by 'culmination' the books of Helena Roerich. Such an interpretation of the words quoted from *Agni Yoga* is confirmed by the following letter of Helena Roerich, where she refers to it as a direct continuation of Blavatsky's teaching: 'Now the Ocean of the Teaching of "Living Ethics" is being given, and whoever has studied it will be equipped for the further path ...'[28] And in another letter she touches upon this question in the following words: 'Anyone who asks what relationship the G[reat] T[eacher] K[ut] H[umi] has to the teaching of "Living Ethics" evidently has no idea what the W[hite] Brotherhood is. Is it really possible that the one Brother [Kut Humi] would reject the teaching given by the other Brother [Mahatma Morya]?'[29]

However, the clearest indication of the source of Helena Roerich's inspiration is the title of the first two volumes of Agni Yoga, published in Paris in 1924–25. They were both called *Leaves of Morya's Garden*, the first book being subtitled *Zov* ('The Call') and the second *Ozaryenie* ('Illumination'). They take the form of a day by day occult diary, in which Helena Roerich has written down what has been imparted to her by her teacher. The first entry is given as 'London, 24 March 1920'.*

Thus we are here concerned with a particular form of mediumistic letter in which the inner 'dictating' voice can be

* According to H.P. Blavatsky her first meeting with Mahatma Morya also took place in London. (See Appendix.)

apprehended by man's day consciousness. The content of the two volumes referred to above corresponds entirely to such a definition. The first contains subject-matter dictated by the teacher in the form of mantric poetry and received in the period between March 1920 and April 1923.

The first London communication begins with the words:

I am your well-being.
I am your smile.
I am your joy.
I am your peace.
I am your strength.
I am your bravery
I am your knowledge
Guard the precious stone, in its unique perfection,
by holiness in life. Aum Tat Sat, Aum.[30]

The whole book is pervaded, as a leitmotiv, by the allegory of an esoteric garden of Eastern wisdom, whose guardian is the teacher guiding Helena Roerich; and the individual utterances are likened to the leaves and flowers that have been gathered in it and which the pupil is instructed to share with other human beings. Some of these are permeated with true poetry, even though their level of thought is for the most part somewhat crude.

Moreover, a mysterious name is constantly repeated in the book: it is denoted by the letter 'M . . .' (with three dots). As the title of the book is *Leaves of Morya's Garden*, the reader is bound to gain the impression that this is who is being spoken of. However, it subsequently emerges that this is another individuality, in whose name and upon whose instruction Helena Roerich's teacher turns to her.

'Give repose to your spirit, do not weary yourself with

books, and love will pour forth in a radiant stream, revealing the wonders of the flowers of M . . .' 'The flowers of M . . . do not prosper in many gardens, but they even blossom in ice-floes', and so on.

Sometimes the 'dictation' takes more direct forms, as when the pronouns and adjectives 'Me' and 'My' – representing the dictating teacher – are written with a capital:

'My lotus is the joy of the visitors to My garden.' 'The fruits and flowers of My garden are accessible to all, be guardians of My garden.' 'But I shall augment the powers of My daughter, for she waits in My garden.' ('My daughter' here means Helena Roerich.)

At times the 'dictation' acquires an openly authoritative form: 'I, I, I read your thoughts every day. The teacher verifies the creative work of his favourite pupils.' Or: 'My smile follows after you, My friends'. And then the same teacher appears almost like a cosmic force:

In the whispering of leaves,
In the lapping of waves,
In the wafting of the wind,
I am with you.

Or:

I am the burning heat of the sand,
I am the flame of the heart,
I am the all-consuming wave,
I am the new-born earth.

And then:

I am a valiant shield,

I teach you My wisdom.
I am not one who promises a bridge but who summons the light!
I teach love.

In some of these pronouncements the 'dictating teacher' is revealed as a member of the mysterious 'White Brotherhood' that lies hidden in inaccessible valleys of the Himalayas: 'Children, children, dear children, do not think that Our Brotherhood is hidden from humanity by impenetrable walls. The snows of the Himalayas which conceal Us do not hinder those who seek in truth.' Or: 'I taught you a happy knowledge, which thaws out the teaching of Tibet'. 'Exhaling fragrance from the mountains of Tibet, We bring to humanity tidings of the new religion of the Pure Spirit.'

The mysterious 'M...' also belongs to this brotherhood, and evidently occupies a central position in it. 'M... has many watch-towers on the slopes of the Himalayas', Helena Roerich's inspirer tells her; and he continues: 'M... teaches you to entreat the pure Brothers that the stages of the mountain path may appear to you'. And then in the form of a command: 'Keep the others true to the ideas of M...' 'Happiness comes to you through the shield of M...' 'Be an Aeolian harp for the wafting of M...' 'Study the manifestations of M...' 'The mountains are clear, M... is with you always.' 'Be bolder, be pupils of M...' 'Follow the teaching of M...', 'M... protects'. 'If you believe Me', continues the inspirer, 'know that you are surrounded by the care and protection of M...', 'M... is your smile, your well-being, your stronghold and knowledge'. And so on. In these and many other pronouncements in the collection, dependence on the teacher as upon a higher divine power becomes truly absolute.

The mysterious significance of the subtitle of the first book, *The Call*, also becomes evident in the relevant statements. 'Do not tarry – M . . . calls.' 'Gird up your strength and open up the path to Me.' Or:

In the forest seek My pointers,
In the mountains listen to My call,
In the murmuring of the stream attend to My
 whispering.

The teacher is always at your door,
But leave your doors open,
Await him and he will answer your call.

The teacher now becomes everything for the pupil, even a father: 'Enter into life in My name and you will conquer the darkness*, for I am your protector, Friend, and Father'. 'I shall set you at My Gates and you will speak in My name. My Word will be with you.'

As we become familiar with this first book of *Agni Yoga* we may well ask: who is this mysterious 'M . . .' of whom the inspirer of Helena Roerich continually speaks? She herself speaks about this inspirer at the beginning of the second volume of *Leaves of Morya's Garden*, 'Illumination': 'People will ask: who gave you this Teaching? Your answer should be: the Mahatma of the East.' This 'mahatma of the East', who – judging by the title of the first two books of *Agni Yoga* – must be Mahatma Morya, then addresses himself to the Roerichs

* These words sound particularly disturbing if they are compared with the following words of Christ: 'I have come in the Name of my Father, and you do not receive me; but if someone else comes in his own name, him you will receive' (John 5:43).

together or apart as 'My children', 'My daughter', 'My son' and so forth. As for the mysterious 'M . . .', in the subsequent volumes of *Agni Yoga* this enigmatic abbreviation is simply replaced by the full name: 'Maitreya'. (However, as there are many places where the reader will not be able to distinguish between Morya and Maitreya, he must come to the conclusion that they are one and the same individuality.)

In the teachings of Agni Yoga he is the 'Great Teacher', the high ruler of Shamballa, where – in the opinion of Helena Roerich – dwell all true mahatmas, for they are the white brothers who usually appear in the dictated material as 'we'. Thus Shamballa is referred to by the dictating agent as 'Our place, Our towers, Our valley, Our mountains, Our stronghold', and so forth. And in the second volume of *Agni Yoga*, *Illumination*, it is described as follows: 'Shamballa is the place where the spiritual world is united with the material. Just as in a magnet there is a point with the greatest power of attraction, so are the gates of the spiritual world open to the Inhabitant of the Mountains.' Nicholas Roerich, too, speaks about the earthly Shamballa hidden somewhere in the depths of the Himalayas, about the mahatmas who live there and its emissaries who work throughout the world, in his article, 'Radiant Shamballa'; this article comes at the beginning of his book, *Shamballa*, which appeared in English (in America) in the year 1930.

The article (of which more will be said later) consists of a long conversation which Nicholas Roerich has about Shamballa with one of the Tibetan lamas during his journey in the Himalayas. Helena Roerich writes more fully about this mysterious land in the second book of *Agni Yoga*, where her inspirer tells her about the various technical achievements that exist amongst the population and in the ashrams of Shamballa, achievements which are as yet unknown to the rest of humanity. Helena Roerich's inspirer tells her about 'our laboratories', to which no one can gain access 'without a call' and 'without a guide'; he speaks of 'our far-seeing apparatuses', 'observatories', 'prismatic mirrors' and so on. According to the inspirer, all this exists somewhere in one of the Himalayan valleys that are inaccessible to human beings.

Later in the same book there is a detailed description of the various kinds of help which the mahatmas of the Himalayan community and its numerous emissaries constantly make available to the rest of humanity in every continent. The influences can be psychic or completely material in nature. Meetings may come about, letters sent or large sums of money – but always from unknown sources. Mysterious unknown figures enter into conversation and give advice to politicians, artists and inventors. Sometimes the mahatmas appear to people physically, and sometimes – to more advanced pupils – in a spirit-body. Finally, only the most advanced are found worthy of a direct introduction – while still in a physical body – to the main 'Himalayan stronghold', to earthly Shamballa, which, according to the Roerichs, is in constant connection with the 'heavenly', or supersensible, Shamballa.

Helena Roerich tells of the 'Teachers of the Gr[eat] Himalayan Community' in one of her letters: 'Never lose sight of the fact that the Mahatma Brotherhood consists of those seven Sublime Spirits who came from the higher planets at the end of the third race [the Lemurian] to hasten the evolution of our humanity. Their spiritual power and their greatness are beyond comparison with any recognised human geniuses...'[31]

In this context, the last, fourteenth and most extensive volume (over four hundred pages long) of *Agni Yoga* – which remained unfinished and was therefore published only after Helena Roerich's death – is particularly characteristic. It consists of five hundred paragraphs, each of which is prefaced by the mahatma who was dictating to her with a direct address to her personally and with a reference to her profound knowledge and highly developed faculties. Moreover, Helena Roerich is throughout called not by her ordinary name but by another, the Indian name 'Urusvati' (which, when translated out of the Sanskrit, means 'Light of the morning star' or 'Light of Venus'). After each such address there follows an explanatory commentary. We shall cite some examples of these addresses: '§1: Urusvati knows the tower Chung [the tower in the Himalayan stronghold where the mahatmas' laboratory is situated]; §4: Urusvati knows how difficult it is to transmit thoughts over a distance; §5: Urusvati has seen Us both in the flesh and in a more refined form; §6: Urusvati can testify to the healing vibrations that are sent forth by Us; §7: Urusvati knows Our voices, both the silent and those that sound; §9: Urusvati has been in Our laboratory; §10: Urusvati knows Our language; §13: Urusvati can speak the Names of the Members of the Brotherhood...; §25: Urusvati has done much to explain why we are called the World Rulership; §31: Urusvati rightly understands the reason for the longevity of Our Manifestations; §48: Urusvati is in constant intercourse with Us;' and so on.[32]

There is no doubt that this five-hundredfold repetition of what is essentially the same formula, by means of which the unknown mahatma – as a voice behind the scenes – affirms the authority of Helena Roerich and the truth of all her communications, is in itself bound to have a powerful suggestive effect upon the reader.

3. The Asiatic Journey of the Roerichs. Conversations with the Mahatmas

The occult significance of the Roerichs' lengthy journey through Mongolia, Tibet and the Himalayas (1925–28) may be better understood if what has been said in the previous chapter is taken into account. The notes which Nicholas Roerich made during the journey are full of examples and stories of various people's meetings with the mahatmas. Summing up these stories, he writes: 'If you cross this remarkable Tibetan plateau with its magnetic waves and extraordinary optical phenomena,* if you hear testimonies of these things and witness them for yourself, you know about the mahatmas. I have no intention of trying to convince anyone of the existence of the mahatmas. Many people have seen them, conversed with them and received letters and material objects from them.'[33] And although the Roerichs only rarely mention their own meetings with the Himalayan mahatmas (in accordance with the strict direction 'not only not to give information about the teachers' whereabouts but not even to speak about it'),[34] nevertheless – as will be apparent from what follows – they had a number of contacts with them.

Several conversations with the mahatmas were subse-

* This is a reference to phenomena such as 'UFOs', the 'Unidentified Flying Objects' which the Roerichs on more than one occasion observed and described during their journeys in the Himalayas. More will be said about their occult origin on p. 79.

quently published in the third volume of *Agni Yoga*. This book, which bears the title *Obshchina* ('Community'), has the sub-title: *Listy besyed vysokovo obshchinnika vostoka* ('Leaves of Conversations of the High Member of the Community of the East'). Here too – as in the first two volumes – the style is couched in the form of direct dictation from one or several Eastern teachers: 'Your books are in our libraries', they tell Helena Roerich; 'do you also have ours? ... Have you read them? ... Greetings [from] the Society of the East!'[35] The notes of the Roerichs' conversations with the mahatmas contained in this volume are at times written in very strange Russian – 'with an Eastern accent', as A. Ter-Hakopyan observes in her foreword, and then she continues: 'Helena Ivanovna [Roerich] is a very fine stylist, but here she wrote as she heard, with all the mistakes, repetitions ... [and] lack of articulation'.[11]*

What, then, did Helena Roerich learn from her inspirers, the Eastern teachers, the inhabitants of earthly Shamballa in the ravines of the Himalayas? Here something most unexpected awaits the reader. In *Community* we read: 'One may ask: "What characteristics do teachers value?" You know the qualities of action and are able to recognise new approaches to action. Preference should be given to that Teacher who follows new paths. In this respect the people of the Northern Land [Russia] have an excellent example – their Teacher Lenin [when referring to Lenin Helena Roerich everywhere without exception uses a capital for the word 'Teacher'] knew the value of new paths. Every word of his preaching, each of his actions, bore the stamp of unforgettable novelty. This difference from other men elicited a compelling power. He

* From *Mozaika Agni-yoga* ('A Mosaic of Agni Yoga'), extracts in two volumes from the 14 volumes of *Agni Yoga*, Tbilisi 1990.

was no imitator, no interpreter, but a mighty moulder of new ore. The summons to innovation should be taken as a foundation.'[36] And then the Eastern mahatmas continue: 'The solidity of his fearless thought forged for Lenin an aureole from both left and right. His firm thinking did not desert him even in illness. His consciousness became concentrated as though in a cave, and instead of discontent and complaint he made remarkable use of his last days. He sent many silent emanations of will for the strengthening of the cause. His last hours were good. Even his last breath he sent to the people. In view of Russia's imperfection, one can accept much on Lenin's account, for there was no one else who could have taken upon himself a greater burden for the general good. It was not because of illness but out of a sense of justice that he even helped the cause of Buddha. And there was no realm that he would have spurned as would many other rulers. His books we love somewhat less, they are too long and what is most valuable about him is not expressed in his books. He did not love his books himself. Lenin is action rather than theory.'

And then there follows something about his cosmic significance: 'Take the phenomenon of Lenin as a sign of the sensitivity of the cosmos ... Let us honour Lenin with our full understanding. Let us show affirmation of the Teacher who maintained a constant inner fire in both success and failure ... When he tore everything down, he created the people's consciousness.' And then all the followers of Agni Yoga are invited to follow the 'leader': 'Lenin thought widely and understood matter. Can you not even to some extent follow the leader?' 'The teacher will be a natural leader. One may rejoice that Lenin is acknowledged to be such a teacher.' 'As pupils of Lenin, watch with the eye of an eagle, and with the leap of a lion claim the power that is yours. Don't miss the boat!'

Finally, the Himalayan mahatmas tell the Roerichs what is of most importance: they speak about their meeting not only with Lenin but also with Marx: 'We know the monolithic way of thinking. We saw Lenin in Switzerland. Our colleague conversed with him in Moscow. He has not changed his views, nor is he unresolved. Everyone knew about the inexhaustibility of his convictions.' And then about the contacts with the founder of Marxism: 'We know the books of Marx and Engels, and our representatives have even spoken with Marx. All their theses can easily be accepted by us. We do not find [in them] anything to ossify or deny matter. It is absurd that the West has not accepted our simple theses, which have been fortified by long experience.' And then one of the mahatmas describes these meetings more fully to Helena Roerich: 'I have already said that our representatives met Marx in London and Lenin in Switzerland. Evidently the word Shamballa was spoken. At different times though independently, both leaders asked: "What are the characteristics of the age of Shamballa?" The answer was: "The age of truth and world community". Both leaders said independently: "May Shamballa come soon." We measure the successors by the words of the leaders. We cannot regard the narrowness of ignorance to be part of Marxism and Leninism. If an ignoramus dares to call himself a Marxist or Leninist, tell him sternly that this is a clear betrayal of the foundations of the community. Do you observe how the word Shamballa is pronounced in the East? Try even if only in a small way to enter into the ideology of this concept. Try to understand the rhythm of the way Shamballa is spoken about, and you will feel the great reality which will make mankind's strings tremble.' Thus somewhere in the very heart of Asia, in the distant Himalayas, the Roerichs were able to learn some curious details about the occult foundations of Marxism-

Leninism and even about its connection with 'Shamballa'.

However, the Roerichs first encountered the Himalayan mahatmas' positive relationship to Bolshevism and its victory in Russia in 1917 not in the Himalayas but seven years earlier in London.

As indicated above, Helena Roerich began to write down the teachings of Agni Yoga – which had their source in the 'dictate' of the mahatmas – in the Anglo-Saxon capital in the spring of 1920. At the same time the Roerichs also began to establish the first groups through which they might be studied. All this activity was the direct consequence of their first direct encounter with the mahatmas on the physical plane, which also took place in London. After this the mahatmas time and again furnished the Roerichs with, as they themselves expressed it, 'material' help. When they again met in the Himalayas, they reminded the Roerichs of this: 'Our community has sometimes been accused of seclusion and of being unwilling to help people. You yourselves know [the true state of affairs], having seen us in London, New York and Sikkim and our colleagues in Moscow.* It is for you to say that we were active as regards outward circumstances and clothing. We learnt in time about needs and new arrivals. You must admit that our London camouflage was resourceful, and our wish to furnish the greatest possible help was remarkable. Our material consignments to Paris and Sikkim were not small. You know that our letters arrive quickly and our messengers are never late. Say this to the young people' (this refers to the members of the Agni Yoga groups founded by the Roerichs).

---

* This probably refers to certain Tibetans who appeared in Petersburg and Moscow at the end of the 19th century and before the Revolution and who tried to make contact with and exercise influence over Nicholas II. (See further in Supplement IV.)

What were the words with which the exposition of the new teaching began, what was the first message of the mahatmas? We find the answer in the very first lines of the first volume of *Leaves of Morya's Garden*, which opens the fourteen-volume series of *Agni Yoga*. This book begins with the following remark on the part of the mahatma: 'My first message for the new Russia'. And then there follows an appeal to Nicholas and Helena Roerich:

> You who have founded an ashram,
> You who have bestowed two lives,* spread the word...

And a promise of protection:

> I shall enclose you with [my] shield – do your work.
> I have spoken.

This command of the mahatma to found the doctrine of Agni Yoga and to propagate it in future above all in 'the new [that is, Bolshevik] Russia' was strictly followed by the Roerichs throughout their lives.† And at the end of their lives they even began seriously to prepare themselves to return to their native land, which, however, proved to be possible only for their eldest son, the orientalist Yuri Roerich, after their death.

This principal aim – the future spreading of the doctrine specifically amongst the Slavic peoples and especially the Russians – was to be furthered not only by the very fact of writing the fourteen volumes of *Agni Yoga* in the Russian language but above all by their particular style, which had

* The Roerichs had two sons.

† See Appendix.

become established from approximately the fourth volume of the series onwards and which – in the minds of those inspiring this work – was intended to correspond to the psychological characteristics of the Russian soul in order to direct its evolution in a certain direction regarded by them as necessary. Agni Yoga could, in its most essential features, be characterised as a purely Eastern doctrine, though in a form adapted for the Slavic soul and psychology.

In connection with the Eastern mahatmas' positive relationship to Bolshevism and, moreover, their part in preparing for the Bolshevik Revolution, the question arises as to the possibility of contacts – even if only of an indirect nature – between them and those secret societies of the West in which the idea of the 'socialist experiment' in Eastern Europe was born in the last quarter of the 19th century.[37] Nicholas Roerich, who lived for many years in America and subsequently visited it several times, meeting there a number of highly placed individuals, was able to serve as an ideal mediator for these contacts.*

The succession of journeys made by the Roerichs to India and America – amongst which the testimony, referred to above, of their meetings with the mahatmas in London, New York and the princedom of Sikkim in North-East India should not be lost sight of – is therefore not without interest. Thus in 1919–20 the Roerichs lived in London, and then between 1920 and 1922 in America, for the most part in New York. From there in 1923 they made their first visit to Sikkim.

* As a rule, the occultists who enter the Western secret societies are in a state of 'secret warfare' with Eastern occultists. However, it seems as though for the purpose of carrying out the socialist experiment first in Russia and then in certain other countries they have managed to reach a compromise and even for a short time – albeit for different reasons – to combine their efforts.

In 1924 the Roerichs were again in New York, where they had no difficulty in gaining permission to undertake the great Himalayan expedition that they were planning under the American flag. Immediately after this, while on the way from America to India, Nicholas Roerich visited the Soviet embassy in Berlin.

The biography of Roerich that was published in 1973 in Moscow speaks at some length about this first direct contact with the official representatives of the Bolshevik government. According to this source, Nicholas Roerich told the Soviet consul about his intimate acquaintance with the mahatmas and those political leaders of India who were opposed to the English colonial powers. In the words which Roerich addressed to the consul, the mahatmas 'believed in the future of Soviet Russia, in its liberating mission, and placed great hopes on it.'[38] In the biography the following further detail is mentioned: 'At Roerich's insistent request, this conversation was recorded verbatim and sent to Moscow', and in response to this there shortly arrived in Berlin the decree of the Bolshevik government that Roerich 'can count on any necessary help from the Soviet authorities'.

There now followed the great three-year expedition of the Roerichs through the Himalayas. It was undertaken under two signs or symbols: the American flag and the tanka of Shamballa bearing the image of the Maitreya Bodhisattva. Every evening both emblems were raised over the camp. The journey itself began and ended with a visit to Sikkim (1925 and 1928). In between there was the unexpected journey of the Roerichs to Moscow, the aims of which will be spoken of below. In Moscow they were paid a visit by the Lichtmanns, the future curators of the Roerich Museum in New York, who had come from the United States especially for the purpose. Shortly after the end of the expedition, the Roerichs again travelled to New York (1929). In 1934 the Roerichs visited America for the last time.*

That Roerich quickly found in North America influential sponsors, patrons and followers, even in circles close to the American government, is evident from the fact of the signing on 15 April 1935 of the Roerich pact for the protection of cultural monuments by President Roosevelt. Moreover, the circle of Roerich's acquaintances in America included President Hoover, the Mayor of New York, J. Walker, the Minister for Agriculture, H. Wallace, the governors of many American states and so on. Roerich's fame is also apparent from the proposal in 1929 to put him forward for the Nobel prize, alongside the then American Secretary of State, the British Prime Minister and an American senator.[39]

As Jacqueline Decter relates in her monograph on Roerich, America also owes it to him that the image of a pyramid appeared on the dollar bank note.†

The question of Nicholas Roerich's possible contacts with those secret societies of the West that Rudolf Steiner speaks of as being the real 'fathers' of the socialist experiment in Eastern Europe[40] must, in the absence of any direct proof, be left open. Nevertheless, all the Roerichs' attempts to unite the ancient spirituality of Tibet and India with the materialism and one-sided scientific and technological progress of the West, whose symbol may rightly be regarded as North America, were only one form of that union of luciferic and ahrimanic powers which appeared in a somewhat different aspect in that socialist experiment to which from 1917 onwards Eastern Europe and subsequently many other countries in various

* In the course of this last journey, certain disagreements emerged between N. Roerich and his American patrons.

† See Supplement V.

parts of the world were subjected.

In 1920 Rudolf Steiner spoke of this as follows: 'What is being attempted [now] in the culture of Eastern Europe? The attempt is being made to exclude everything of a truly human nature that is embodied in human corporeality and to harness Lucifer and Ahriman together in their distinctive culture. If this were to be brought about today in the East [of Europe], the fruits of the combined activity of Lucifer and Ahriman would make themselves manifest, thereby excluding everything that can benefit the human individual – who would then be thrust into this luciferic and ahrimanic culture as a component of a machine is incorporated into this machine, except that, whereas the component of a machine is lifeless and allows itself to be thus incorporated, human nature is inwardly alive and imbued with soul and spirit, and hence, being unsuited to a purely luciferic and ahrimanic organisation, must perish in it.'[41]

And no amount of calls on the part of the Roerichs in the name of humanity and of a caring attitude towards earthly culture and historical monuments can do anything to change this true state of affairs.

4. The Roerichs' Mission to Bolshevik Russia

The brief visit made by the Roerichs to Moscow in 1926, for the sake of which they interrupted their Himalayan expedition for a short while, acquires a particular significance in the context of our present considerations. This journey was made by them at the direct indication of the mahatmas and had as its aim the fulfilment of one important task assigned by them to the Roerichs. In essence, this consisted of the following.

The trans-Himalayan expedition began in March 1925 from Kashmir, in North-West India, whither the Roerichs had come directly from Sikkim where they had had meetings with the mahatmas. During their stay in Kashmir the Roerichs made an intensive study of the collection of legends and traditions according to which Jesus Christ did not die in Palestine on the Cross but was rescued and miraculously brought to the Himalayas by his spirit-teacher Chitan Natkhye, under whose instruction he had been in the period between his fourteenth and thirtieth years. Thereafter he lived for several years in Kashmir and died there. On his grave, which is still there today, the inscription can be read: 'Here lies Issa [Jesus], son of Joseph'. The extent to which the Roerichs took these legends seriously is apparent from N. Roerich's picture on this theme entitled 'Issa and the Giant's Head'. It depicts a solitary figure with a halo around his head, which in outline is supposed to be reminiscent of Jesus contemplating a gigantic skull belonging to a giant in one of the valleys in the Himalayas.*

From Kashmir the expedition moved on northwards through the Western Himalayas. It was on this section of the journey that – according to what is said by the mahatmas – the third volume of *Agni Yoga*, *Community*, was written, although it is possible that its content originated in the meetings at Sikkim. Moreover, the mahatmas now gave the Roerichs the wholly concrete commission of visiting Moscow and bringing their letter to the Bolshevik Government and the consecrated Himalayan earth to Lenin's grave. In fulfilment of the mahatmas' commission, the Roerichs directed their expedition – together with the letters and gifts – towards the Russian border and by 13 February were in Kashgar, which lies not far from it. There immediately followed a visit to the Soviet consulate and an intensive study of Soviet newspapers, under which impression Helena Roerich wrote in a letter: 'With great enthusiasm we read "Izvestiya" – what a magnificent project – and were especially moved by the veneration with which the teacher's name – Lenin – is surrounded ... This is indeed a new country, and the Dawning Light of the Teacher shines brightly over it ...'[42] In the next big town, Urumchi, the Roerichs stayed several weeks waiting for their Soviet visas. Every evening they went to the Soviet consulate and read the consul excerpts from their book *Community* about the

* See Supplement VII. In 1988, a book came out in Srinigar (India) by the Kashmir historian F. Chassanaiya entitled *Fifth Gospel*, where the testimonies, legends and traditions about Jesus' time in India before and after his three year period of activity in Palestine are collected. In his book the Indian scholar claims that the principal source for his research was a Tibetan manuscript discovered in 1925 by the Russian artist Nicholas Roerich. (See the compendium entitled *India*, the article Jesus Christ and India: Legends and Tales', Moscow 1991.)

mahatmas' relationship to Lenin and the Bolshevik Revolution.[43] For Lenin's birthday Nicholas Roerich, at the consul's request, in one night made a sketch for the pedestal of the bust of the 'leader' (newly brought from Moscow). This little episode merits particular attention, not only as yet another testimony of the Roerichs' veneration for the Bolshevik founder of 'the new Russia' but also for another reason. Thus in one of the biographies of Roerich it is described as follows: 'During the artist's stay in Urumchi a bust of Lenin was brought from Moscow to be displayed in front of the consulate building. As there was no pedestal for it, Nikolai Konstantinovich had prepared a sketch for one to be erected. However, after one of his visits to the consulate Roerich wrote in his diary: "... the truncated pyramid looks somewhat forlorn – like the pedestal of a forbidden monument. It is impossible to understand that, while all placards of Lenin are allowed and the Chinese drink for the prosperity of Lenin's cause, his bust cannot stand on a pedestal that has been prepared for it". Meanwhile the displaying of the bust was forbidden on the personal orders of Yan Dutu [the Chinese Governor-General of this province of China].'[44]*

The interesting point in this episode is the detail of the *form of the pedestal* as conceived by Roerich: a *truncated pyramid* with Lenin's head placed upon it. This form crops up again later in Roerich's life. In 1935, during his third and final visit to America, he gave the American state officials – through his friends – the idea of portraying a truncated pyramid on the one dollar note (see p. 31). Thus to this very day the design of these notes incorporates a *truncated pyramid*, on which, however, is placed not the head of Lenin but a triangle with the image of an eye, that is, the ancient symbol of the Father God,

* In the 1920s China was not yet communist.

the great Creator of the Universe. But there can be hardly anyone in America who is now aware whose image Roerich had intended to crown *his* 'truncated pyramid'.

The visa eventually arrived and the Roerichs could now leave for Moscow by train via Omsk. Moreover, together with their permission to enter Bolshevik Russia there also came – evidently from central sources – a special instruction to the OGPU (which was what the KGB was called in the twenties) to help the Roerichs in every possible way on their journey to Moscow and to work with them.

In connection with this circumstance, Roerich noted in his diary: '9 June [1926], Omsk: We go to the OGPU to leave our weapons for safe-keeping. Again that same courtesy and solicitude. "How can we help?" 10 June: We are on our way The train leaves at midnight. The OGPU gave the order that we be helped to find our seats ... At midnight the train [Omsk-Moscow] arrives. The OGPU agent goes past and indicates with his eyes that all is well.'[45] Just imagine the improbability of the situation! An expedition, journeying through Asia with secret aims, departing from an English Colony under the American flag,* 'in the official documents' of whose members it is mentioned that they were making 'for Moscow as the mahatmas' special representatives, to fulfil their commission'†, was permitted by the Bolshevik Government to enter Soviet Russia unhindered, and then just as freely allowed to leave the country, and, moreover, in the direction chosen by the participants themselves. All this can only be explained if the 'representatives of the mahatmas' and their

* In Jacqueline Decter's monograph there is a photograph of the camp of the Roerichs' Asiatic expedition, with a big American flag unfurled over it.
† V. Sidorov. See note 3 to the Appendix.

'letter' were taken far more seriously in the Kremlin than it might appear at a first glance.

In the capital they were officially received by two members of the Bolshevik Government – the People's Commissar for Foreign Affairs, G. Chicherin, and the People's Commissar for Education, A. Lunacharsky. In the course of a conversation of many hours with them, Roerich spoke at some length of 'the possibility of uniting Russia and the great world of Buddhism with the help of the Mahatmas',[46] and gave Chicherin a casket from them containing the consecrated Himalayan earth and the letter.

'Half communist and half Buddhist', was how Chicherin described Roerich after the conversation. And in their letter the mahatmas write: 'We are sending the earth for the grave of our brother Mahatma Lenin'. 'In the Himalayas we know what you have accomplished. You have abolished the church, which had become a breeding-ground of falsehood and superstition. You have wiped out the bourgeoisie, the source of prejudice. You have destroyed the prison of education. You have rooted out the seeds of hypocrisy. You have consumed the army of slaves with fire. You have crushed the spiders of profiteering. You have shut the gates of the dark dens of vice. You have liberated the earth from treacherous embezzlers. You have recognised that religion is the teaching of the all-embracing nature of matter. You have recognised the insignificance of personal property. You have discovered the key to the evolution of society. You have indicated the significance of knowledge. You have bowed down before Beauty. You have brought children the full might of the Cosmos. You have opened the windows of the palaces. You have seen the urgency of building new houses for the common good.'

Then the mahatmas go on to speak about their own cause: 'We stopped an insurrection in India that was premature, we also recognised the timeliness of your movement and send you our help, thus affirming the Oneness of Asia. We know how much will happen in the years 1928–31–36. We greet you, who seek the Common Good!'[47]*

In addition to the gifts of the mahatmas, Rocrich also presented the Bolshevik Government with gifts of his own. He gave to Lunacharsky a cycle of seven pictures under the general title of 'Maitreya', and also a large canvas entitled 'The time has come', where over a peaceful Earth there appears the head of a giant bogatyr [knight] gazing towards the East, in whose face the features of Lenin are easily recognisable.[48] The artist defined the idea of the picture as follows: 'The time has come for the peoples of the East to awaken from their age-old sleep, to throw off the chains of slavery', which, in his opinion, is to come about through the rapid spread of Bolshevism from Russia throughout the whole of Asia.

We shall now dwell at greater length upon the message of the mahatmas that was written in 1925 and endeavour to single out its most important elements. There are three. Firstly, the elevation of Lenin to the rank of mahatma and the allusion to the help afforded by the mahatmas to the Bolshevik Revolution of 1917 and the subsequent establishing in Russia of Bolshevik power and ideology: 'we send You our help'.

Secondly, the prophetic allusion to the years 1928–31–36, in which period the Bolsheviks, under Stalin's leadership,

---

* In connection with this letter of the mahatmas to the Bolshevik Government, as with their indications contained in H. Roerich's letters to the American President, F.D. Roosevelt (see Supplement V), one question remains unresolved: were these letters given to the Roerichs in a ready, written form, or dictated by the mahatmas when they met, or communicated to them in a mediumistic way through occult dictation, as with all the volumes of *Agni Yoga*?

made the transition to total terror. 1928 – the preparation and beginning of forced collectivisation, which was associated with the wholesale annihilation of the peasantry; 1931 – the process of industrialisation grips the entire country, gradually transforming it into a vast labour-camp; 1936 – the beginning of mass terror, which reached its peak in 1937, when millions of innocent people were without trial or investigation shot or sent away to camps (the so-called first wave of mass Stalinist repressions).

Finally, the third and perhaps most significant element. In the letter the following words are addressed to the Bolsheviks: 'You have recognised that religion is the teaching of the all-embracing nature of matter'.

In order that we may better understand this very strange 'revelation' of the mahatmas, it is necessary to turn to other, still stranger, 'revelations' as contained in the book *Community*. There the Himalayan mahatmas tell Helena Roerich: 'Collectivism and dialectivism* are two aids to thinking about materialism. The nature of materialism has a particular mobility, and does not fail to encompass any of life's phenomena. The teacher merely lays down the necessary landmarks. It is possible to develop principles for this manner of thinking. Materialism must become established to such a degree that all the scientific achievements of modern times are able to enter constructively into the understanding of it. We have spoken about astral bodies, magnets, the radiance of the aura, the emanation of every object, the shift of sensibilities, the change in gravitational forces, the penetration of one layer of matter by another, the sending of thoughts through space, the phenomenon of the cementing of space, the feeling of

* Meaning 'dialectic'. The word was incorrectly written by Helena Roerich.

centres, the understanding of the word matter. Much that is invisible and discernible only by apparatuses must be grasped by one who wishes to introduce technology into life. It is necessary to replace idealistic blather by solid reasoning power. *We materialists* have the right to demand the respect and recognition of matter.'[49] 'Childish materialism is a narcotic for the people, but the materialism of enlightened knowledge will be a ladder to victory.'

And then, probably recalling their meetings with Lenin in Switzerland, the mahatmas continue: 'We have already seen how a communist receives the teaching. We have already seen how easy it is to speak with a communist. For one we are mahatmas, for another we are scholars, for a third rebels, for a fourth a committee of revolutionaries, but the teaching itself encompasses all the hopes of the communists. Our conditions for colleagueship are a total wish to apply our principles to life, not theory but practice.' And in this connection there is talk of the need to 'give instruction regarding the material nature of thinking'.

Then the mahatmas go on to say: 'You rightly think that technology is impossible without communism ... as *practical materialists* we can boldly assert this'. These words have much in common with a well-known aphorism of Lenin: 'Communism is Soviet power plus the electrification of the whole country', which served as the basis for turning the entire country into a giant labour camp.

The mahatmas view the future age of the Maitreya (the age of Aquarius) in the same way: 'The Buddha has incorporated himself as a man, as the Teacher of affirmation. In this leonine, fiery affirmativeness he has attained to a preview of the Maitreya – *the age of the knowledge of the greatness of matter.* Affirm matter in all its manifoldness and oneness!' Thus 'in the teaching of the Buddha we find not only materialistic philosophy but the practical improvement of each day . . . Never do we call the Buddha meek, for on the contrary he is an intrepid leader, a fighter for community and matter, a hero of labour and unity.'

In these and many other places in *Community* one may be astonished by this mixture of Bolshevik terminology and Buddhist ideas. For example, there is the following observation in *Community* about the first two volumes of *Agni Yoga*: 'If your thinking is not yet purified by the true hammer and sickle*, take up the book *Illumination* and the book *The Call*.' Or: 'One who wishes to devote himself to true communism acts in accordance with the principles of great matter'. And then the mahatmas explain quite openly: 'Those who have understood reality and materialism can ally themselves with our community. It is impossible to think of a mystic or metaphysician as being behind our walls.' 'Communism, supported by technology, gives a mighty spur to knowledge.' And all this they call 'the ideology of Shamballa'.

The consequences of the mahatmas' indications in *Community* regarding pedagogy and practical work with children are particularly dire, if one bears in mind that such work is being carried out today in many 'Roerich groups'.

The following utterances of the mahatmas in *Community* can give a certain impression of their 'pedagogical ideas': 'It is necessary to examine the programmes of schools and strengthen the quota of materially reliable knowledge. The idealism of superstition drives people into abysses of horror. It is necessary to carry out this rectification of educational thinking with alacrity, otherwise yet another generation of

* The 'hammer and sickle' were the chief symbols of the Bolsheviks, and were incorporated in the emblem of Soviet Russia.

imbeciles will disgrace the planet. Natural science must be strengthened, once the significance of this work has been understood. Biology, astrophysics and chemistry draw the attention of the youngest child's brain. Give children the opportunity to think!'

And in another context: 'The education of the people must be introduced at the earliest possible age from the first lesson. The sooner the better. Be assured that an overstraining of the brain happens only through clumsiness. Every mother who approaches a child's cradle will express the first educational formula: You can do everything ... The awareness that "I can do everything" is not vainglory but merely a matter of becoming aware of the apparatus.'

The mahatmas demand as much abstract, intellectual knowledge as possible at a very early age. The sooner it is begun the better. Of particular importance is the work with children *before the age of three*, for 'only a consciousness of below the age of three is readily receptive to the community'.

In these quotations we have a complete contrast to the basic principles of the pedagogy founded upon the anthroposophical view of man, according to which it is not right to overburden a child with intellectual knowledge at an early age (especially before the age of three), since this makes the future adult particularly prone to ahrimanic influences (materialism). From the point of view of anthroposophical pedagogy children do not only have a physical brain that needs developing but are beings with a threefold spirit and soul organism, which must be developed in its entirety.[50]

We shall confine ourselves to these quotations, which could be multiplied without any difficulty. Later on we shall examine the occult foundations of this remarkable devotion of the Himalayan mahatmas to Bolshevism. Meanwhile we need merely to observe that the mahatmas' acknowledgement of the central significance of materialism is by no means simply a 'discovery' on the part of Helena Roerich. For similar utterances can be found in a book already mentioned in these pages, *The Mahatma Letters to A.P. Sinnett.* These were letters received by the English journalist from the two theosophical mahatmas Kut Humi and Morya, with whom he had entered into contact through Blavatsky.

One such extract from a letter of one of the mahatmas (Kut Humi), where he himself imparts the foundations of the teaching of the Himalayan mahatmas about matter, is quoted in the letters of Helena Roerich. The reason why she quotes the mahatma and tries to defend his views is not without interest. Helena Roerich's letter is an answer to a letter from one of her pupils, who was troubled by the avowed materialism and even atheism contained in the mahatmas' teachings. Before answering her correspondent, Helena Roerich first once again quotes the portion of the mahatma's letter in question, having previously – as she says – verified it with the English original*: 'Then you refer to the *deeply philosophical* statement of the Elder Mahatma: "As to God – since no one has ever or at any time seen him or it – *unless he or it is the very essence and nature of this boundless eternal matter, its energy and motion*, we cannot regard him as either eternal or infinite or yet self-existing. We refuse to admit a being or an existence of which we know absolutely nothing, because ... there is no room for him in the presence of that matter whose undeniable properties and qualities we know thoroughly well ... In other words, we believe in *matter* alone, in matter as visible nature and matter in its invisibility as the invisible omnipresent omnipotent Proteus ..." '[51]

* The italics are in the original letter. A fuller extract from the letter is reproduced in Supplement VIII.

These words of the mahatma appear in a letter sent by him to Sinnett in 1882. And in 1934 Helena Roerich tries to defend this as follows: 'You are disturbed by this glorifying of matter. But do you not know that in esotericism matter and spirit are one? That matter is merely a differentiation of spirit? Do you not know that matter is also energy, for one does not exist without the other? ... Do you not know that Spirit, bereft of matter, does not have phenomenal form, in other words, does not exist? Indeed, in our actions and thoughts we cannot separate ourselves from matter. We are dealing with either the higher levels or the baser aspects of the same matter.' (The last two phrases are a quotation from *Community*).[52]

And in another letter, again responding to the same objections, Helena Roerich adds: 'Matter or the most refined substance of Spirit-Matter is infinite in its differentiations and in its visible and invisible manifestations, but it is impossible to do anything with pure spirit. Ignorance separates and analyses everything, but the Great knowledge of the East unifies and synthesises everything.'[53]

From these quotations there unfolds a remarkable sequence in the activity of the mahatmas, from Blavatsky and Sinnett to Helena Roerich and her Agni Yoga.

In the following words, Helena Roerich speaks about the significance of the mahatma letters to A.P. Sinnett and their connection with the chief work of Blavatsky, on the one hand, and the teachings of 'Living Ethics' on the other: 'But it is useless and erroneous to condemn and deny the "Letters of the Mahatmas". Sinnett's *Esoteric Buddhism* was based on these "Letters". Their content – developed further – led to [Blavatsky's] *Secret Doctrine*. The volume of these "Letters" is a very great book, and it is highly esteemed in the West. To deny it means to deny the whole teaching that was given through Blavatsky and also all the books of "Living Ethics".'[54]*

But let us return to the Roerichs. Once he had discharged one commission of the mahatmas in Moscow, Nicholas Roerich immediately made it known to the members of the Ministry for Foreign Affairs that he had to return to India at once – and, moreover, via Mongolia – in order, as he said, to fulfil there further 'commissions of the mahatmas'.[55]

Whether because of the magic effect of the word 'mahatma' or for other reasons, the Roerichs obtained permission for their departure from Bolshevik Russia through Mongolia and China almost directly. As for the special mission entrusted to them in Mongolia, it was most probably in some way connected with the anonymous publication in the Mongolian capital, Ulan-Bator, of two books by Helena Roerich: *The Foundations of Buddhism* and the third volume of *Agni Yoga, Community*, with all the above-quoted utterances of the mahatmas about Lenin, communism, the Bolshevik Revolution and so forth. Without doubt these publications, which rested on the authority of the mahatmas, were to serve to further strengthen and extend the power of Bolshevism in Mongolia and China.

To be sure, Mongolia had by then already been under Bolshevism for three years. The Bolshevik revolution there was carried out in 1924 by Sukhe-Bator, who had previously visited Lenin in the Kremlin. The results of the revolution was the destruction of all seven hundred Buddhist monasteries on Mongolian territory and also the killing or the incarcerating in camps of over a hundred thousand Buddhist monks. In his

* Helena Roerich subsequently translated a portion of these letters into Russian and published them under the pseudonym of Iskander Hanum in 1925. (See Supplement VIII.)

writings, Nicholas Roerich points out that the Mongolian soldier-revolutionaries were singing this song on the streets of Ulan-Bator (its words were written by Sukhe-Bator):

The war of Northern Shamballa.*
Let us die in this war
To be reborn again
As Knights of the Ruler of Shamballa.

Nor did Nicholas Roerich stand aside from these events. Before leaving Mongolia he presented its Bolshevik government with the picture 'The Great Horseman' – painted in the traditional Mongolian style – which depicted 'The Ruler of Shamballa – the Maitreya', with the assembly of the 'Great Khural' (the higher organ of power in Bolshevik Mongolia) portrayed in its lower part. In presenting this picture to the leader of the Mongolian government, Tserendorzh, Roerich explained: 'The Mongolian people is building its radiant future under the banner of a new age. The Great Horseman of liberation is sweeping over the Mongolian expanses ... And loudly sounds the call of the *red*, beauteous Kingly Horseman [the Maitreya].'

In answer to these words, Tserendorzh – who had visited Lenin together with Sukhe-Bator, on the eve of the Mongolian revolution – said the following: 'May the idea of our common teacher Lenin spread throughout the world like the flame in this picture, and may the men who follow this teaching continue their work with the same sense of resolution with which the Great Horseman portrayed here gallops

* By 'Northern Shamballa' is meant Bolshevik Russia. Roerich often employs this name for Russia in his books. See, for example, his *Heart of Asia* and *Shamballa.*

on his way.'[56] As a result the Roerichs received from the Mongolian government a charter of protection for their further expedition.

Now the Roerichs' path led through Central Tibet back to India. The arduous expedition, in the course of which they had to cross several high passes with heights of up to 5000 metres, came to an end in May 1928 in the place where it had started: in the princedom of Sikkim in North-West India, which was where Mahatma Morya had visited Blavatsky.* [57] The Roerichs had spent two years here before the beginning of the expedition (1924–25). Moreover, it was here that the idea of it had been born, and where their own meeting with the mahatmas had taken place (see the quotation on p. 27). Now, on returning there, Nicholas Roerich founds his institute of Himalayan research 'Urusvati', which means 'Light of the morning star' or 'Light of Venus', a name which was at the same time the title given by the mahatmas to Helena Roerich (see p. 22), who was chosen as its first and life-long founder-president. In December 1928 the Roerichs again leave Sikkim and eventually settle in Kulu in North-West India, whither the institute for Himalayan research is also transferred. Henceforth and until their death, Kulu in Kashmir becomes their principal place of residence.

Nevertheless, the Roerichs' positive attitude to Bolshevism and to all the 'successes' of the Russian people in building their 'radiant future' remained unchanged in subsequent years.

---

* In connection with this Nicholas Roerich wrote the following in his diary during his first visit to Sikkim in 1923: 'There was in Sikkim one of the ashrams of the mahatmas. In Sikkim the mahatmas journeyed on mountain ponies. Their physical presence has endowed these places with a solemn significance. Of course, the ashram has now been moved from Sikkim. The mahatmas have, of course, left Sikkim. But they were here.'

Thus Helena Roerich wrote in one of her letters in 1935: 'Our fatherland has set out upon a path of recovery and seeks a new and glorious path. The most gratifying symptom is that the masses have awoken to conscious life...'[58]

Similar thoughts can also be found expressed by Nicholas Roerich. In 1940 he wrote: 'The Russian people have piled together great stones. To the admiration of everyone they have built no tower of Babel but a Russian tower. A Kremlin of Sun-bearers with a hundred towers!... Listen – that is the future, and how radiant it is!'[59] Or in 1941: 'The whole world is rushing towards Armageddon. Everyone is confused. Everyone is unsure about the future. But the Russian people have found their course and with a mighty flood are streaming towards their radiant future.'[60] And in 1943 he counsels: 'May the Leninists remember the legacy of dialectical materialism,'[61] and so on.

Indeed, the Roerichs remained to the end faithful to the precepts of the Himalayan mahatmas. Moreover, this deep devotion to the East was even expressed in Nicholas Roerich's outward appearance; for towards the end of his life – despite all his Russian and Swedish ancestors – strongly Asiatic and Mongoloid features appeared in his face, just as happened in the case of him whom he and his inspirers so admired, 'Mahatma Lenin'.

5. The Occult Foundations of the Teachings of Agni Yoga

Now that we have characterised certain aspects of the outer activity of the Roerichs and the teaching given through Helena Roerich, we must consider its occult foundations from an anthroposophical standpoint. In the first place we need to turn to the highly surprising fact of the deeply positive attitude of the Himalayan mahatmas to Bolshevism. There is doubtlessly a connection between this fact and their secret meetings with Marx in London and with Lenin in Switzerland, their pronouncement of the latter as a 'mahatma' and also their occult and political support of the Bolshevik Revolution of 1917 and of the subsequent rule of the Bolsheviks, of which they wrote in their letter to the Soviet government, and so on.

The attitude of the present-day followers of the Roerichs in Russia to this letter of the mahatmas is not without interest. Thus, for example, V. Sidorov, the President of the Commission for the Literary Heritage of Nicholas Roerich, writes in the foreword to the reprint of the first – Ulan-Bator – edition of *Community* published in 1990 in Moscow: '[The message of the mahatmas] opened up a possibility unprecedented in history: to make what was considered a legend into a real fact of politics. After all, the authors of the message were mahatmas, mysterious and – as it were – mythical beings. And now came the suggestion to establish regular contact with them and even to depend on their support.'[62]

Whence came this evident interest on the part of the

Eastern mahatmas in the victory and spread of Bolshevism not only in Russia and Asia but throughout the Earth? Rudolf Steiner gives a very clear and simple answer to this question out of the sources of anthroposophical spiritual-scientific research: 'For these Eastern initiates the results of Leninism do not contain anything terrible, for these initiates say to themselves: If these institutions of Leninism are spread ever more widely over the Earth, this will be the surest way of bringing doom to earthly civilisation. But this will work to the benefit of precisely those people who through their previous incarnations have created for themselves the possibility of carrying their existence forward without the Earth.'[63] Helena Roerich comforts her followers in a similar vein. In her opinion, 'all who are truly devoted to knowledge of the light [by which she means Agni Yoga] and the common good will [in the event of the Earth's extinction] go on to higher planets. Sad will be the lot only of those who are left behind fluttering around the fragments of the disintegrated boat [the Earth] or who have departed to Saturn.'[64]

In the above-quoted words of the spirit-researcher who derives his knowledge from modern Christian initiation, we have a clear indication of the sources of inspiration of these Eastern initiates or mahatmas. For the endeavour to draw humanity away from the Earth *before* its earthly mission – as is made manifest through a true knowledge and a realising of all the impulses springing from the Mystery of Golgotha – has been fulfilled is the central task of Lucifer with respect to earthly evolution as a whole. And that cosmic kingdom, in which alone a humanity that has been deprived of the Earth will be able to live, will be Lucifer's realm.

In other words, the chief inspirers of the Eastern mahatmas in their efforts to attain this goal are luciferic spirits. This is also the source of the deep antipathy to Christianity with which

Blavatsky had been inspired by the mahatmas, and of the unconditional devotion to Lucifer as 'the great benefactor of mankind' (see Rudolf Steiner's words quoted on p. 12). It is true that in Helena Roerich's letters it is possible to find not infrequent references to Lucifer as an evil, negative spirit. However, these references actually relate to Ahriman, whom Helena Roerich always calls Lucifer. This is made especially evident by her reference to the fall of Lucifer in the fourth root race, on Atlantis,[65] that is, in that period of earthly evolution when the ahrimanic spirits first entered into the evolution of humanity.[66] Moreover, in those same letters Helena Roerich describes 'Lucifer' or 'Satan', who tempted man in paradise and thereby endowed him with the gift of distinguishing between good and evil, as the great benefactor of humanity, 'since this gift could *not* be given by the power of darkness but was sacrificially bestowed by the Forces of Light. Hence the original name of this Emissary was Lucifer, the Light-bearer.'[67]

Thus as the knowledge of Christ, who brings the true balance between Ahriman's forces of darkness and Lucifer's one-sided forces of light, was inaccessible to Helena Roerich, the whole teaching of Agni Yoga is drawn into the opposition between these two categories of spiritual beings, which in many of her letters is characterised as the battle between the powers of light and the powers of darkness (also called Armageddon).

However, this does not mean that we do not also find in Agni Yoga a significant ahrimanic influence. This is manifested with the greatest intensity in its teachings about matter and in its *occult materialism.* Already in the Himalayan mahatmas' letters of 1926 to the Bolshevik government they openly declare their support and agreement with the following proposition of 'scientific materialism': 'You have recognised that religion is the teaching of the all-embracing nature of matter'. 'We are materialists'; 'we are practical materialists', declare the mahatmas in the third book of *Agni Yoga, Community*.

To the whole series of similar utterances of the mahatmas cited on p. 39, we shall add here one further remark which is particularly characteristic: 'Accept it when people call you materialists. In our thoughts and actions we cannot separate ourselves from matter. We are dealing with either the higher levels or the baser aspects of the same matter.'[68] However, similar ideas had lived in various forms within the Theosophical Society since the time of Blavatsky, when, for example, the wholly supersensible etheric body was conceived of as being similar to the physical, as simply being composed of 'more refined matter' or 'higher vibrations',[69] completely forgetting that the real transition from matter to spirit is not of a quantative but of a *qualitative* nature. Rudolf Steiner indicated several times in his lectures that such notions of the supersensible are the residue of modern materialism. 'But everywhere in the universe where there is ether is emptier than empty. That is why it so hard for physicists to speak about the ether, because they always think that ether is also matter, only more rarefied, more so than ordinary matter. This idea about more rarefied conditions of matter is entertained both by scientific and theosophical materialism; the conception is of ever further stages of rarefication. First there is dense matter; etheric matter is more rarefied, astral matter still more so, and then there are all these mental states of matter and everything to do with them – ever more rarefied [material] conditions. Such ideas are entertained just as much by theosophical as by scientific materialism, except that the former enumerates more stages of rarefication [of matter] than the latter. But the transition from ordinary weighable, ponderous matter to the ether has nothing to do with becoming more rarefied.' (Later in the same lecture Rudolf Steiner fully characterises what this transition is from a spiritual-scientific point of view.)[70] Further such 'residues' of materialism are the altogether false conception of certain theosophists regarding the 'permanent atom' which, as they would have it, passes as a constant particle of matter from one incarnation to another and so on.[71] This very evident inclination towards materialism, as we have seen, already appears in the mahatmas' letters to Sinnett. 'We believe only in matter...', wrote the mahatma Kut Humi in one of these (see p. 43). And Helena Roerich wholly logically draws the following conclusion in her teachings from this proposition of the mahatmas: 'Outside matter, pure spirit is a nothing.'[72]

In order to understand this at first apparently so strange mixture of Eastern spirituality and Western materialism, which in 1907 Rudolf Steiner called a 'barren hybrid', it is necessary to turn once more to the anthroposophical teaching about the eighth sphere and to dwell upon certain aspects of it.

According to Rudolf Steiner's spiritual-scientific research, the arising of the eighth sphere around the Earth is connected with the *combined* activity of Lucifer and Ahriman, who, while being irreconcilable opponents on one level of world existence, can, nevertheless, on another level be entirely successful in uniting their efforts, as is indicated in the left-hand motif of the Sculptural Group.* This combined activity of theirs led to

* In the nine-metre high Sculptural Group, which depicts Christ overcoming Lucifer and Ahriman, there is a lateral motif where both spirits of opposition are shown combining their forces against the right evolution of mankind. The Sculptural Group was intended for the First Goetheanum, which was burnt down in 1922. It is at present in the Second Goetheanum.

the gradual arising of the eighth sphere, which as regards its essential nature does not belong to any of the seven spheres, or planetary stages of development, through which man passes in the course of the complete cycle of world evolution from Saturn to Vulcan. Initially it arose through Lucifer – who always longs to conserve the past stage of earthly evolution with the aim of illicitly leading it over to the next stage – introducing into the present Earth evolution the forces of Old Moon, which in their original form can only be perceived in visionary, atavistic clairvoyance.

The Old Moon was formed in such a way that the higher spiritual worlds and their laws were continually reflected in its spiritual sphere as in a mirror; and it was through the permeation of Moon evolution by these reflections that Old Moon had by the end of its evolutionary cycle come to be transformed into the 'planet of wisdom', which then, after passing through a pralaya, served as the foundation of the modern Earth. It is this supersensible substance of Old Moon, containing in itself the imaginative reflection of the higher worlds, that Lucifer now illicitly introduces into earthly evolution. Here, however, he is joined by Ahriman, who endeavours to wrest from the Earth sphere the dense, physical matter which has been legitimately formed within it and is connected only with its evolution in order to impregnate it with the cosmic imaginations preserved by Lucifer from Old Moon. These Moon imaginations which have been thus densified by earthly matter form the content of the eighth sphere.

'Thus', says Rudolf Steiner, 'we are enclosed in a world of densified imaginations, which are not Moon imaginations for the simple reason that they are densified by the material element of the Earth. But they are spectres – that is, behind our world is a world of spectres created by Lucifer and Ahriman

... Thus into our fourth earthly sphere has been incorporated a sphere which is really a Moon sphere but which is wholly filled with the earthly material element [i.e. matter], and is, therefore, an utterly false phenomenon in the universe.'[73] Rudolf Steiner goes on to speak about the goals which the opposing forces seek to attain with the help of the eighth sphere: 'According to the intentions of Lucifer and Ahriman, nothing less than the disappearance of the whole of human evolution into the eighth sphere is a prospect for humanity, as a result of which its entire evolution would have to take a different course.'[74]

In order that this should not happen, the Spirits of Form (Elohim) who guide earthly evolution sent one of their number, Jahve or Jehovah, to the Moon, which he gradually permeated with such dense matter that Lucifer and Ahriman were unable to draw it away with them into the eighth sphere. Thus Jahve became mankind's great defender from the forces of the eighth sphere, for he 'took pains to ensure in the physical domain that not the whole of the material realm could be sucked away by Lucifer and Ahriman [into the eighth sphere].' In this sense the spreading of Sinnett's false assertions that the Moon, which has the task of opposing the eighth sphere, represents this very sphere, and also Blavatsky's teachings, with her veneration of Lucifer and her negative attitude towards Jahve and Christ, were to a significant degree intended to further the development of 'occult materialism' amongst mankind (see p. 9).

In such an 'occult materialism' something similar takes place on the human plane, in the sphere of knowledge, to what the opposing forces bring about together on a cosmic plane substantially, in real existence, in order to strengthen the eighth sphere: Lucifer brings the imaginations of Old Moon, and Ahriman permeates them with earthly matter. And as these Moon imaginations, as has been shown, contain the reflections of higher spiritual worlds, through their being permeated by earthly matter these higher worlds themselves begin to appear to a human individual who beholds them in the reflections of the eighth sphere as though they are permeated by ever more refined matter. Thus Agni Yoga teaches: 'We are dealing with either the higher levels or the baser aspects of the same matter' and 'outside matter, pure spirit is a nothing'. Such utterances can indeed spring only from inspirations from the eighth sphere.

All this enables us to understand more clearly a further thesis of Agni Yoga (*Leaves of Morya's Garden vol. 2, Illumination*): 'Astral bodies have volume and weight and possess many of the qualities of earthly life'.[75] Behind such a statement lies the following reality: If a human individual begins to develop an inclination towards occult materialism during his life, after the death of such a person Lucifer acquires the possibility of bringing part of his astral body into the eighth sphere, and Ahriman of impregnating this astral body with earthly matter. In this new spectral existence it then actually acquires certain attributes of the physical world, 'volume and weight', as it were.

From what has been said it becomes more possible to understand the significance of the union in the books of Sinnett and Blavatsky between Eastern esotericism and Western materialistic science. In an occult sense this union is none other than the concrete expression of the combined activity of Lucifer and Ahriman in the process of creating and strengthening the eighth sphere. This trend is directly continued in Agni Yoga, which – in the words of its founder – aspires to find 'connecting links between the ancient traditions of the Vedas and the formulas of Einstein.'[76] The architecture of the Roerich Museum in New York was to become a visible symbol of these 'connecting links'. The artist himself conceived it in the form of a 24-storey skyscraper, crowned by a round Buddhist stupa.

6. The Principal Error of Agni Yoga

Now that we have, with the help of Anthroposophy, considered the occult foundations of Agni Yoga's devotion to Bolshevism and materialism, we must turn to the central error of this teaching, to its inability to recognise the Christ Being and His whole significance for world evolution. This lack of understanding can be traced directly to the Eastern mahatmas who inspired Helena Roerich and whose initiation Rudolf Steiner described as follows: 'The Eastern initiations must necessarily leave the *Christ principle*, the central *cosmic* factor of evolution, untouched.'[77] From an esoteric point of view this inner blindness with regard to a true understanding of the Being of the Christ stems from the fact that the spiritual experience of the Eastern initiates extends only to the lunar and planetary spheres and not to that of the Sun. This means that their occult knowledge embraces only the world of the planets which make up our solar system, and 'the higher *planetary spirits*' which rule them – 'the only "spirits" we believe in', write the mahatmas.[78] As for the Sun, the spiritual focus of our cosmic world, it is perceived by them merely in its lower, 'planetary' aspect, that is, as an integral *part* of the solar system and not as a mediator for, and a gate into, the higher spiritual worlds lying beyond it, which in an occult sense corresponds to the higher aspect of the Sun not as a 'planet' but as a 'star'.[79]

The Eastern mahatmas give indications of this limitation in their knowledge to what is *within the bounds of the solar system* on several occasions in their letters to Sinnett and other theosophists. Thus the mahatma Kut Humi writes: 'You were told that our knowledge was limited to this our solar system'.* And then in another letter: 'What lies beyond and outside the worlds of form, and being, in worlds and spheres in their most spiritualised state ... is useless for anyone to search after, since even Planetary Spirits have no knowledge or perception of it. If our greatest adepts [of the East] and Bodhisattvas have never penetrated themselves beyond our solar system ...'[80] And in another letter: 'No adept has ever penetrated beyond the veil of primitive Cosmic matter. The highest, the most perfect vision is limited to the universe of *Form* and *Matter.*' And finally in yet another letter: 'Not even a Dyan Chohan of the lower orders could approach it without having its *body* consumed, or rather annihilated. Only the highest "planetary" can scan it'.[81] Despite the overtly materialistic character of the later statement, it follows clearly that for the Eastern mahatmas direct access to the inner *Mysteries of the Sun*, to its deepest, 'starry' secrets, remains closed. Thus their higher occult knowledge is confined to what can be received by initiates who in their spiritual development have risen to the Bodhisattva stage, that is, beings 'who have never penetrated themselves beyond our solar system'.

The Christ Being is at an opposite pole to the Bodhisattvas. Whereas a Bodhisattva is a highly developed *human being*†, Christ is a cosmic divine Being. In other words, whereas a

* See Supplement VIII.

† The human nature of the Buddha was acknowledged in the Theosophical Society. Its co-founder, Olcott, for example, expressed this in a short Buddhist catechism which he compiled for schools in Southern India. While in her foreword to *The Foundations of Buddhism* (in Russian), Helena Roerich wrote: 'The great Gautama gave the world a complete teaching of life. All attempts to make the great evolutionist into a god lead to absurdity.'

Bodhisattva, in becoming a Buddha, ascends to the outer limits of the solar system, that is, to the 'mantle' of the starry Mysteries of the Sun, Christ, as a higher divine-cosmic Being, *descends* from the worlds lying beyond its bounds, uniting first with the higher 'starry' aspect of the Sun and then with its planetary aspect, in order from thence to descend to Earth for the fulfilment of the central Event of earthly evolution – the Mystery of Golgotha.[82] Thus from the sources of Christian initiation Rudolf Steiner speaks about Him as follows: 'Christ, Who now reveals Himself as the Being who at the beginning of our era passed through the Mystery of Golgotha, *descended to the Sun from still greater heights*'.[83]

At the boundary between the 'starry' and 'planetary' aspects of the Sun a meeting takes place between the descending Christ and the ascending Bodhisattvas, who together form there a high spiritual lodge, with Christ representing the central Sun, or starry, principle and the Bodhisattvas the planetary or Moon principle. For, just as the Moon reflects sunlight, transmitting it from itself to the Earth, so do the Bodhisattvas receive in this exalted sphere, and then bring to all mankind, the light and knowledge of the central Being of our cosmos, its spiritual Sun – the Christ.

Rudolf Steiner unfolded this highly important mystery of esoteric Christianity from the sources of Christian-Rosicrucian initiation. In a whole series of lectures given in 1909–10 he referred to the circle of twelve Bodhisattvas who in the sphere of Buddhi or Providence surround the higher source of their inspirations, their knowledge and their life – the Cosmic Christ: 'Thus to Christ there belong twelve Bodhisattvas, who have the task of preparing and further establishing what He [the Christ] has brought as the greatest impulse of our cultural development ... By this means we have risen to the sphere of the Bodhisattvas and have entered a circle of twelve stars with the Sun at its centre, illuminating and warming them. This Sun is as that source of life which they will then bring down again to the Earth.' This is the true relationship between Christ and the Bodhisattvas: 'Christ at the centre of earthly evolution, and the Bodhisattvas as His predecessors and successors, who have the task of renewing humanity's relationship with His work.'[84] Thus in another lecture Rudolf Steiner calls the Bodhisattvas the 'emissaries of the Moon (lunar sphere)' or, which is the same thing, the 'representatives of the 'Moon Logos', which in the spiritual spheres of the Moon and the planets is 'the reflection of the Sun Logos' or the Christ.[85]

However, this aspect of the activity of all *true* Bodhisattvas remains completely closed to the Eastern mahatmas, with the result that they apparently know nothing of their higher aim of serving the Sun Logos – the central Being of our cosmos, Who on one single occasion became flesh in Jesus of Nazareth.* This 'becoming flesh of the Logos' (John 1–14) opened up to earthly humanity for the first time in its whole existence the possibility of gaining *direct* knowledge of the most hidden essence of the Sun mysteries in their higher, 'starry' aspect – which unites our solar system with the entire universe, extending even to the regions of the highest spirituality, that is, those divine-spiritual worlds which are in Chrisitan esotericism rightly called the worlds or kingdom of the Divine Father – not through the mediation of the Bodhisattvas, that is, not through the reflection of the Sun Logos by the lunar Logos (as was the case in pre-Christian religions), but from the

---

* In the thick volume of the mahatmas' letters to Sinnett, with its 500 pages of small script, letters which form the basis not only of his book *Esoteric Buddhism* but also of Blavatsky's book *The Secret Doctrine*, Christ is not mentioned at all.

Christ Himself, Who passed through the Mystery of Golgotha and has since that time been united with the whole of earthly evolution.* Herein lies the esoteric significance of Christ's words: 'No one has ever seen God; the only-begotten Son, Who is in the bosom of the Father, He has made Him known' (John 1:18). In other words: the mysteries of the spiritual cosmos lying beyond our solar system were not accessible to any of the Earth's initiates until the coming of Christ. Now, however, through union with the Christ impulse, they have become accessible to all who follow the path of Christian initiation.

In our time the revelation of these Sun Mysteries of the Christ takes place in Anthroposophy. Through his knowledge of them Rudolf Steiner, as the modern Christian initiate, was in a position to penetrate in his spiritual research into the evolution of our solar sytem not only to the limits of the Earth aeon but also to the limits of the aeon which proceeded it, that of the Moon, and to the aeons of ancient Sun and ancient Saturn – of which Eastern wisdom knows virtually nothing.† Thus everything that the Eastern mahatmas were able to dictate to Sinnett and Blavatsky, especially in *The Secret Doctrine*, remains almost entirely within these limits: 'By far the greater part of what was given by Helena Petrovna Blavatsky in *The Secret Doctrine* is derived from this consciousness which reaches back only to ancient Moon. This is known by all occultists who have investigated these matters. Thus if you study *The Secret Doctrine*, you will find in its great, all-

* 'Lo, I am with you always, until the closing of the age' (Matthew 28:20).

† Knowledge of these is attainable for Eastern wisdom only indirectly, through their microcosmic repetition at the very beginning of the Earth aeon (see GA 13 and 11).

encompassing panorama of primal beginnings precious little about a more distant past than the [ancient] Moon condition, which preceded the present Earth condition.'[86]

In this sense, what Rudolf Steiner imparted in his book *Occult Science* about the two more ancient cosmic conditions, and also about the three future aeons of world evolution, those of Jupiter, Venus and Vulcan, represented a truly colossal step forward. Rudolf Steiner subsequently spoke about this as follows: 'So when – this was between 1906 and 1909 – in my book *Occult Science* I described the Earth in its earlier incorporation of ancient Moon, in its still earlier incorporation of ancient Sun and finally in its earliest incorporation of ancient Saturn, you will see that I did not stop at its incorporation of ancient Moon but went further back to the condition of ancient Saturn;*[87] whereas all the initiates who spoke about these matters came to a halt between Moon and Sun and, hence, went back only to the Moon sphere.† They became uninterested and even at times disturbed if it were suggested that they look further back into the past. They declared this to be impossible, for there one encounters a barrier, *in the form of a veil*, beyond which one cannot penetrate.'[88]

These words of Rudolf Steiner have a remarkable amount in common with the following passage from a letter of the mahatma Kut Humi (September 1882), where he similarly speaks of the 'veil' which forms the limit of the 'correct' knowledge of the mahatmas: 'So far – We KNOW. *Within* and to the utmost limit, to the very edge of the cosmic veil we

---

* In the lecture of 31 October 1911 Rudolf Steiner speaks of how in the course of his spiritual research he was able to reach the sources of existence of the very first aeon of our cosmos, that of Saturn, only because he 'was borne by the Christ Being', 'felt at one with the Christ Being'.

† As is clear from the context of this lecture, this refers mainly to the *Eastern* initiates standing behind and inspiring Blavatsky.

know the fact to be correct – owing to personal experience; for the information gathered as to what takes place beyond we are indebted to the planetary spirits, to our blessed Lord Buddha. This of course may be regarded as second-hand information.'[89]

Modern Christian-Rosicrucian initiation, however, makes it possible for this 'information' to be received at *first* hand. In the lecture of 13 April 1912 Rudolf Steiner fully characterises the relationship of Gautama Buddha to the Planetary Spirit of Mercury who inspires him* and then to Christ. Here, too, there is on the one hand the ascent of the spiritual consciousness of Gautama – when he became a Buddha – to the sphere of the Planetary Spirit of Mercury, who in his turn serves still more exalted Sun Spirits belonging to the 'starry' aspect of the Sun, and on the other hand the descent of the Cosmic Being of the Christ through the upper, 'starry' gates of the Sun, first to the sphere of the higher Sun Spirits, that is, the rulers of the *entire* solar system as a single entity, and then to the sphere of the Spirit-rulers of the individual planets. On this level the Cosmic Christ, as the Ruler of the entire Kingdom of the Sun amidst the Planetary Spirits who serve Him, is like a radiant Sun encircled by the choir of the planets; and this is repeated nearer the Earth, when Christ appears not only to the Planetary Spirits but also to the Bodhisattvas who are guided by them, and who contemplate and serve the Cosmic Christ as was described above.

Thus in characterising Buddha's relationship to Christ at the end of the lecture referred to above, Rudolf Steiner says: 'When Blavatsky identified Buddha with Mercury, she was expressing a profound truth which can be better understood

* In *The Secret Doctrine* Blavatsky – or, rather, her inspirer – refers to the existence of this connection between Buddha and Mercury.

to the extent that one grasps the relationship of Buddha to Christ in the occult sphere, just as cosmic relationships are best understood if one comprehends the relationship of the planet Mercury to the fixed star of the Sun. These things cannot be dismissed from view out of human prejudice; for they can work rightly in the cultural process only if we confront them directly and in an unbiased way.'[90] In these words Rudolf Steiner is referring to the endeavour of Blavatsky and other theosophists to place Buddhism higher than Christianity, and Buddha higher than Christ – which is ultimately based upon a complete ignorance of the true Christian Mysteries. For Eastern initiation affords access only to an understanding of beings of the rank of Bodhisattva and Buddha and also of the higher Planetary Spirits who guide them, whereas the Mysteries of the Cosmic Christ, the Sun Logos Who rules our cosmos, remain completely beyond its ken. 'The Eastern initiations', writes Rudolf Steiner, 'must necessarily leave the *Christ principle*, the central *cosmic* factor of evolution, untouched'.[91]

However, precisely because it is impossible for the Eastern initiates to comprehend Christ's true nature, any real relationship to His coming to the Earth – and that of 'the blessed Lord Buddha', whom they revere above all other adepts – is also barred to them. Hence they know nothing of how the latter, having attained the position of the highest honour and now abiding in the supersensible body of the Nirmanakaya, was at the beginning of the Christian era working in the astral body of Jesus of Nazareth, preparing his sheaths for receiving the Sun Logos, the Christ, at the Baptism by John in the Jordan. For this mystery of the *further evolution of the Buddha* in the supersensible worlds – after his last earthly incarnation in the 6th century BC – is accessible only to the Mysteries of Christianity. Similarly, the true relationship of Gautama Buddha to the highest earthly guardian of these mysteries,

Christian Rosenkreutz, remains an enigma for them (see further below).

Rudolf Steiner has the following to say about Gautama Buddha's participation in the events of Palestine out of the sources of the modern Christian mysteries: 'The oriental tradition is right to assert that Buddha was born as a "Bodhisattva" and that he rose to the rank of Buddha only during his earthly life, in his twenty-ninth year. When Gautama Buddha was still a little child, the Indian sage Asita came weeping into the royal palace belonging to Buddha's father. This was because he was – being clairvoyant – able to know that this king's son would become the Buddha and because, as an old man, he would not live to see Suddhadana's son attain this rank. This sage was born again in the time of Jesus of Nazareth. He it was whom the Gospel of St Luke portrayed as the priest of the temple who saw Buddha revealed in the ... Jesus child. And seeing this he said: "Lord, now lettest thou thy servant depart in peace, for I have seen my Teacher!" What he had not been able to see before in India he saw now through the astral body of this Jesus boy who comes before us in St Luke's Gospel: the Boddhisattva who became the Buddha. All this was necessary in order that the body which was subsequently to receive the Baptism by John in the Jordan might come into being.'[92]

In the book from which this quotation is taken, and also in many of his lectures, Rudolf Steiner speaks at some length about the additional participation of other great initiates and teachers of humanity in the preparation of this central Event of earthly evolution – the incarnation on Earth of the Sun Logos and His passage through the death and Resurrection on Golgotha, an event which signified the beginning of a new world epoch and laid the foundations of a completely new relationship of the Earth and humanity with the whole spiritual cosmos.

Since this time it has been the principal task of true Rosicrucians to unfold the entire earthly and cosmic significance of this central Event to all people of good will. Rosicrucians work in the world out of the direct inspirations of Christ, Who is served in the supersensible worlds not only by all true Bodhisattvas but also by all Planetary Spirits (provided they are not of a luciferic nature*). For, in Rudolf Steiner's words, 'the deepest purpose of Rosicrucianism is to reveal ... the intentions of the *living Christ* ... in a form that is filled with wisdom, beauty and active strength'.[93] Thus only 'those who have understood that the future progress of humanity depends upon an understanding of the great Event of Golgotha are they who have united as the Masters of wisdom and of the harmony of feelings in the great ruling lodge of mankind',[94] the spiritual focus of the true White Brotherhood.

These masters of esoteric Christianity (at whose head stands Christian Rosenkreutz), who have in the deepest sense understood the full cosmic significance of the Christ impulse and the Mystery of Golgotha, were the inspirers of the modern science of the spirit, or Anthroposophy, founded by Rudolf Steiner at the beginning of the 20th century, the principal task of which is to make the true knowledge of Christ accessible to the whole of mankind.[95]

It follows from this that one would seek in vain for a true knowledge of the Christian mysteries from either the Eastern mahatmas or from Blavatsky, who was under their influence. Rudolf Steiner says in this connection: 'The mystery of Sinai and Golgotha is not to be found in Madame Blavatsky, for she had a real antipathy towards it. Consequently, she was led towards such forces as were able – and with great power and

---

★ In the lecture of 13 April 1912 quoted above, Rudolf Steiner also speaks about retarded, luciferic Planetary Spirits.

clarity – to give what lay outside Christianity.'[96] 'From this arose *The Secret Doctrine*, which with regard to everything that is not Christian contains great truths, but with regard to everything that is Christian contains nothing but utter nonsense.'[97] This same tendency is also visible in Helena Roerich. Not for nothing does she in her letters and books emphasise in every way possible her inner devotedness to her Russian predecessor: 'I tell you, H.P. Blavatsky was a fiery messenger of the White Brotherhood', she writes in one of her letters; 'she was in a quite particular way a bearer of the knowledge entrusted to it. Of all theosophists only H.P. Blavatsky had the good fortune to receive the teaching directly from the Great Teachers in one of Their Ashrams in Tibet ... Only through H.P. Blavatsky was it possible to approach the White Brotherhood, for she was a link in the hierarchic Chain ... For the good of the cause, the Mahatmas corresponded with some of her colleagues [for example, with Sinnett], but none [save Blavatsky] did they admit to pupilship ... H.P. Blavatsky was that hierarchic link whom to avoid or disregard would have signified total failure.'[98] And in another letter Helena Roerich describes how Blavatsky after her three years in the ashram with the mahatmas 'was sent' by them 'into the world to give the great work *The Secret Doctrine* in order to bring about a change in the consciousness of a humanity that has arrived at an impasse',[99] that is, to give something to the world in which a new and completely Eastern orientation of the entire theosophical movement – which is to say, its anti-Christian aspect – appears clearly.

In connection with Blavatsky, Helena Roerich refers very frequently also to her own association with one of her (Blavatsky's) teachers, Mahatma Morya. Thus in a letter of 23 October 1936 she writes: 'I know that Mahatma M[orya] was not satisfied with all the biographies written about

Bl[avatsky].' Or in a letter of 22 June 1936 she recalls: 'In [19]25 [that is, just before the Roerichs' journey to Bolshevik Russia at the behest of the mahatmas], it was indicated to N[icholas] K[onstantinovich Roerich] that he should paint the picture 'The Messenger' and donate it for the founding of the Bl[avatsky] Museum. Through this gift and the founding of the museum the Gr[eat] Teacher M[orya] wished to perpetuate the name of her whose memory some of her successors have recently been trying to suppress.'[100] This picture was apparently painted in Sikkim, where the Roerichs were staying at the time (cf. p. 27 and p. 47).

But let us return to the underlying question posed above regarding the relationship of the teaching of Agni Yoga inspired by the Eastern mahatmas to the Christ impulse. Quotations from the Gospels and references to the Founder of Christianity are met with fairly often in Helena Roerich's books and letters. This fact is often cited by her followers as proof of Agni Yoga's positive relationship to Christianity. However, if one examines such instances more carefully it immediately becomes obvious that Christ is regarded there merely as one of the many teachers of humanity, of the same rank as Gautama Buddha. For example, in a letter of 24 May 1936 Helena Roerich writes: 'You are right that Jesus [Christ] is a remarkable phenomenon in history, but one should add that all the Kumaras and God-men were no less remarkable. And only a conceited ignoramus will begin to weigh up which of these sublime Spirits is higher or lower. For an excellent formula has been given us in the Teaching:* If the question arises as to who is higher, Christ or Buddha, answer

* By 'teaching' here is meant the books of *Agni Yoga* written by Helena Roerich. Objectifying it in this way is indicative that the content of these books originates not from her but from the mahatmas who dictated to her.

that it is impossible to measure the distant worlds, we can only take delight in their glory'(*Leaves of Morya's Garden vol. 2, Illumination*).[101]

However, this vague definition is given only for the outer, exoteric world. In her correspondence with her esoteric pupils Helena Roerich expresses herself far more clearly. Thus in a letter of 24 September 1935, again after referring to the words quoted above from the *Leaves of Morya's Garden*, Helena Roerich elucidates them as follows: 'Indeed, Christ and Buddha are such distant stars of the spirit in comparison with us earthly [people]. Let us not forget that They and the Lord Maitreya came from Venus*[102] at the dawn of the birth of physical man, and are hence our Divine Forefathers and Teachers.'[103] In these words is expressed the underlying conviction of Agni Yoga, that the Maitreya, Gautama Buddha and Christ belong to the same level of development and that all three came to the Earth from Venus during Ancient Lemuria. And in another letter, where she characterises the 'future epoch of the Maitreya', Helena Roerich again asserts the equality of all three 'Teachers': 'The future epoch will stand under the rays of the Three Lords – the Maitreya, the Buddha and the Christ.'[104]

From the standpoint of Christian esotericism, however, the only element in these words which corresponds to the truth is the indication that the Buddha originally came from Venus. Nevertheless, in the light of Rudolf Steiner's spiritual-scien-

---

* Helena Roerich conceives of Venus in a highly fantastic and materialistic way, as a kind of upgraded version of the Earth. In a letter of 13 August 1938, drawing either upon the mahatmas or Blavatsky's *Secret Doctrine*, she writes about it as follows: 'It is said that on higher planets there are fewer animals and that they are far more perfect. Thus on Venus there are no insects or beasts of prey at all. People fly, birds fly and even fish. Moreover, the birds understand human speech...' and so on.

tific research even this fact has a completely different significance and different causes. For after the separation of Venus and Mercury from the Sun, Christ, the Sun Logos and sublime Ruler of the Sun Kingdom, sent the future Gautama Buddha as His messenger first to Venus and from thence to the Earth: 'The Christ first sent him [the future Buddha] to Venus . . . Thus you have in the Buddha an old emissary of the Christ, who had the task of preparing for Christ's work on the Earth.'[105] 'This individuality of the [future Gautama] Buddha had already been sent from the Sun, from the hosts of Christ, to the Venus men before they – as is recounted in my *Occult Science*★ – returned to the Earth, so that that individuality which lived in Buddha was Christ's messenger from the Sun to Venus. He [the future Gautama Buddha] descended to the Earth with the Venus men; but because of the circumstances indicated he so outstripped the other [men] that during Atlantean times and on into the post-Atlantean age he was able to develop to Buddhahood, attaining this stage before Christ's appearance on the Earth. He was, so to speak, a Christian before Christ . . . Accept this result [of occult research], that Buddha was an emissary of the Christ and as such initially lived on Venus.'[106] The Bodhisattva who in the distant future will reach the stage of Buddhahood and, as the new Maitreya Buddha, 'will become the bearer of goodness . . . and will place his words of goodness at the service of the Christ impulse, is to a still greater degree a pupil and follower of the Christ.'[107]

★ What is meant here is the former period of Earth evolution – described in *Occult Science* – in the course of which it was impossible to find on Earth suitable bodies for incarnation and many human souls were forced to seek further possibilities of evolution on other planets of the solar system (including Venus). Subsequently, when the conditions on Earth had reverted to a more favourable aspect, they again returned to it.

On the basis of these words we may characterise Gautama Buddha as the last preparer of Christ's incarnation on the Earth, and the Maitreya Buddha as His greatest earthly successor, as the first Christian Bodhisattva, who already in our time has as his chief mission that of serving the Christ and 'renewing humanity's relationship with His work'. (More will be said about the modern mission of this Bodhisattva later on.)

That this mystery of the relationship between Christ and the Bodhisattvas was known to Rudolf Steiner from the very beginning of his activity as a teacher of Christian esotericism is evident from the fact that one of his first lecture-cycles, given before he became the leader of the German section of the Theosophical Society, bore the title, 'From Buddha to Christ' (twenty-four lectures given between October 1901 and March 1902). In his autobiography, *The Course of My Life*, Rudolf Steiner writes in recollection of this: 'In these lectures I tried to show what an immense advance the Mystery of Golgotha represents in comparison to the Buddha event and how the evolution of humanity, in that it aspires towards the Christ Event, arrives at its culmination.'[108]

As for Helena Roerich, access to these truly central mysteries of earthly evolution remained closed to her, as it remained closed to her Eastern inspirers. In this sense, those words with which Rudolf Steiner characterises the relationship to these mysteries of her Russian predecessor can also be applied to her: 'And so it happened that Madame Blavatsky was increasingly compelled to experience a mist gathering around her [as regards the true knowledge of Christ], and was able clearly to see only what had been transmitted through so-called purely Aryan traditions ... outside the domain of Christianity.'[109]

We shall cite here one characteristic example. In the second volume of *Agni Yoga* the following description can be found:

'. . . The star of Allagabada* pointed the way, and so we visited Sarnat and Gaia. Everywhere we found a mockery of religion. On the way back, at New Moon, a memorable saying of Christ's was expressed. During the night's expedition the leader lost his way. After some searching I found Christ sitting on a sandy hillock, looking at the Moon-spangled sand. I said: "We have lost our way, we must look to the positions of the stars". "Rossul Morya, what is the way to us when the whole of the Earth is waiting for us. . . ?" Taking a bamboo cane, he drew a square around the impression of his footprint, and added: "Verily I say – a human foot". Then, making a print with his palm, he enclosed it with a square. "Verily I say – a human hand". Between the squares he drew some similarly shaped columns and covered them as it were with a hemisphere. He said: "O, how Aum will enter into human consciousness! There, I have drawn a pistil with an arc above it, and have created a foundation for it with four sides. When the Temple where my pistil is blossoming has been built with human feet and human hands, may the builders follow my path. Why do we wait to find a path when it lies before us?" Then he stood up, erasing with the cane what he had drawn.'[110]

This extract from *Agni Yoga*, where Mahatma Morya gives an account of his meeting with Christ, was illustrated by Nicholas Roerich in 1924. In his painting the seated figure of Christ (the face is not visible, and there is no halo) is portrayed with his back to the spectator, and behind him, though at the same time as it were towering *over* him, is the larger figure of the seated Morya, covered from head to foot by a cloak from beneath which only the sharp outlines of a nose and a dark beard are visible. Both figures are bending over the drawing

* Allagabada is a town in Southern Nepal, on the Ganges.

described above on the earth. The figure of Christ is pointing at it with a small cane and is evidently already preparing to 'erase what he had drawn'. The picture bears the title, 'The Signs of Christ'.

The places mentioned in the passage cited here lie not far from Sikkim and are associated with the earthly life of the Buddha. The Roerichs visited them at the end of 1923. In his diary Nicholas Roerich makes the following observations in this connection: 'Sarnat and Gaia – places associated with personal exploits of the Buddha – lie in ruins. They are merely places of pilgrimage, just as Jerusalem is not more than a place of pilgrimage to Christ . . .'[111]

Whether this description has a bearing on the Kashmir legends about Christ-Issa's stay in India after his flight from Palestine, or – which is more likely – has to do with a contemporary meeting of Mahatma Morya with the Founder of Christianity, now reincarnated and concealed somewhere in the Himalayas, is left wholly unclear.

One thing is certain: despite the complete failure of the Krishnamurti episode at the beginning of our century, the idea of physical incarnations of Christ – both in the past and the future – was one that neither Helena Roerich nor her inspirers were able to renounce. But from the standpoint of Christian esotericism, to speak of any physical incarnations of Christ either before or after the Mystery of Golgotha signifies a complete misunderstanding of the essential nature of the Christ impulse, upon whose fulfilment depends the entire future of the Earth.

7. Some Conclusions

The inner blindness of Agni Yoga towards the spiritual sphere of Christ that we have characterised is manifested with particular clarity in one of its central teachings, that about Shamballa. Its foundations are contained in Nicholas Roerich's conversation with the Tibetan lama. This was published in the article 'Radiant Shamballa', in which Roerich clearly distinguishes between two aspects of Shamballa, the earthly and the heavenly. Addressing the lama he says: 'Lama, we know the majesty of Shamballa. We know that this is indeed an indescribable kingdom. But we also know of the reality of earthly Shamballa. We know that certain high lamas went to Shamballa, and that on their way they saw familiar physical objects. We know stories about the Buryat lama, that he was led by a very narrow secret path. We know that a fellow traveller saw a caravan of mountain-folk with salt from the lakes on the border of Shamballa. Moreover, we have ourselves seen the white frontier post of one of the three frontiers of Shamballa. So do not speak with me only about the heavenly Shamballa but also about the earthly Shamballa; for you know just as well as I that the earthly Shamballa is connected with the heavenly Shamballa. And by means of this link both worlds are united.'[112]

In the books of *Agni Yoga* and her letters, Helena Roerich has a lot to say about the earthly Shamballa, which is also called the 'Trans-Himalayan Stronghold' or the 'Stronghold of Light' and is situated somewhere in one of the inaccessible valleys of the Himalayan mountains. According to her testimony, the earthly Shamballa – now led by the Bodhisattva Maitreya – is the hidden abode of that secret 'community' where all the mahatmas live in physical and 'refined' bodies. From there they visited H.P. Blavatsky, and from there they wrote the letters to her and to Sinnett which were to form the foundation of their books. In a letter of 23 July 1936 Helena Roerich writes about the way to it: 'Many miles from that town [she is referring to one of the towns in Tibet] lies the Stronghold of Light. The approaches to this stronghold are well guarded. There are various ways to it, and it is often necessary to follow subterranean paths and go under rivers in order to reach the hidden heights. But there are landmarks for those who have been called.'[113] Or in another letter : 'The Himalayan Mahatmas live in total seclusion and admit into their Stronghold one, or at the most two, candidates in a century.'[114] In this same letter, the Mahatmas Kut Humi and Morya are named as inhabitants of this 'stronghold'.

According to Helena Roerich, Appolonius of Tyana,[115] Paracelsus[116] and the Count of Saint-Germain[117] were formerly in the 'Trans-Himalayan Stronghold'. From this same 'spiritual sanctuary in the heart of Asia' there also worked the mysterious Prester John, the last guardian of the Holy Grail.[118] Furthermore, in one of the ashrams of the 'Trans-Himalayan Stronghold' H.P. Blavatsky was prepared for the writing of her book *The Secret Doctrine*. Helena Roerich writes of her: 'Sometimes the Mahatmas summon brethren for a certain time to one of their Ashrams and prepare their organisms for [otherwise] hidden perceptions of refined energies and give them instructions. Thus it was in the case of H.P. Blavatsky, who spent three years in their Ashram before sending *The Secret Doctrine* out into the world',[119] and so on.

The extent to which these and similar communications on the part of Helena Roerich may be questionable is shown very clearly by her own allusion to the subsequent spiritual destiny of Blavatsky. Thus, responding in one of her letters to the suggestion that she might be a reincarnation of Blavatsky, Helena Roerich writes: 'But I assure you that I am *not* a reincarnation of H.P.B. She whom they [the theosophists] awaited [H.P. Blavatsky] incarnated around forty years ago and in 1924 safely arrived in the physical body in the main Stronghold';[120] and in another letter she explains that Blavatsky, 'who almost immediately after her death reincarnated in Hungary, has been living in the physical body at the main Stronghold for almost ten years and is now working for the salvation of the world under the name of Brother X.'[121]

Hence in Helena Roerich's opinion, Blavatsky, who died in 1891, reincarnated on the Earth at the end of the 19th century and in 1924 was in earthly Shamballa in the Himalayas. This assertion, however, is in complete contradiction with Rudolf Steiner's spiritual research, according to which the soul of the founder of the theosophical movement was still in the spiritual world between death and a new birth in 1910–12. Thus in a whole series of lectures Rudolf Steiner refers to the importance for Blavatsky's after-death existence of correcting the errors that she had made on Earth as quickly as possible, and particularly all those which had sprung from her complete misunderstanding of and negative attitude towards the Christ impulse. For example, in the lecture of 8 May 1910, which was dedicated to the 'day of the white lotus', that is, the festival of Blavatsky's birthday in the Theosophical Society, Rudolf Steiner says: 'Thus in H.P. Blavatsky we see the bringer of a new dawning light. But what good would that light be if it had no wish to illumine the most important thing that mankind has ever had? A theosophy which does not have the means to understand Christianity [and Blavatsky's theosophy was of such a kind] has absolutely no value for the culture of today.'[122] And then Rudolf Steiner goes on to say that those of Blavatsky's followers who reject the true knowledge of Christianity 'impede the activity of her spirit in our age! ... This spirit is now working in the spiritual world...'[123] Finally, in the lecture of 27 September 1911, where he characterises Blavatsky's transition from the Rosicrucian inspirations lying at the foundation of *Isis Unveiled* to the Eastern and the fundamentally anti-Christian *Secret Doctrine*, Rudolf Steiner adds: 'That this is said is precisely what H.P. Blavatsky, who is not in incarnation now, would wish'.[124] Also in the lecture of 8 May 1912, Blavatsky is spoken of as 'being today in the spiritual world'.[125]

But let us return to the characterisation that Helena Roerich herself gives of earthly Shamballa or the 'Trans-Himalayan Stronghold'. As has already been mentioned, she depicts this secret realm in a highly materially real way. Thus in the second volume of *Agni Yoga* (*Leaves of Morya's Garden, vol. 2, Illumination*), the mahatmas tell her about 'our laboratories and observatories',[126] our 'prismatic mirrors', 'our telescopic apparatuses'.[127] And in a letter of 24 June 1935 Helena Roerich mentions 'an apparatus that collects psychic energy' and 'apparatuses which measure the tension of the fire of space',[128] and adds: 'All these apparatuses work not only on a refined level but also on the physical plane in the Fortress of the Great Brotherhood'.[129]

In all these and similar descriptions, which are repeated again and again in the pages of *Agni Yoga*, we encounter in a sense a kind of spectre of the eighth sphere: all the 'visions' of Helena Roerich are hopelessly impregnated by the conceptions of modern materialistic science and appear in a highly material form. It is possible that this is associated with the fact that during the great Himalayan journey (1925–28) the Roerichs continually encountered phenomena in the mountains of which little was known or spoken about at that time but which have since the middle of our century become accessible to many hundreds of people in various continents and have received the name of 'unidentified flying objects'. In his book on Shamballa Nicholas Roerich recalls the 'remarkable plateau of Tibet with its magnetic waves and miracles of light'.[130] And in another article he himself reports to the Tibetan lama: 'Lama, not far from Ulan-Davana [a place near the Northern border of Tibet] we saw an enormous dark vulture ... it crossed the path of something radiant and beautiful which was moving southwards over our camp and shining in the rays of the Sun. The lama's eyes lit up: "O, Shamballa is protecting you ... the protective power of Shamballa is accompanying you in the aspect of this Radiant Matter ... Did you notice the direction in which this sphere was moving?"'[131]

What the Roerichs on several occasions observed in the twenties in the Himalayas and is now observable throughout the world in the form of 'flying saucers' has in fact nothing to do with the true Shamballa but has its origin in the eighth sphere, which since the middle of our century has been strengthened and densified to such an extent that its phenomena have become accessible to an ever growing number of people. Luciferised imaginations of Old Moon, which in their original form can be apprehended only through imaginative consciousness, are permeated to such an extent by matter that has been wrested from earthly evolution and has been taken hold of by Ahriman that they become visible to man's outward, physical sight in the form of hallucinations.

Rudolf Steiner characterises this combined work of Lucifer and Ahriman in the following words: 'Ahriman interferes with our perception of outer phenomena and deceives us with regard to them. Nevertheless, we could unmask his intentions if Lucifer did not awaken certain inner longings and incite us towards such materialistic notions in our view of the world.'[132] And then Rudolf Steiner indicates in connection with these processes that the principal source of the matter which the opposing forces are continually trying to gain mastery over in order to draw it into the eighth sphere is the human head, the human brain, the most perfect and spiritualised part of the physical body. Thus when people think only materialistic thoughts, as is currently the case for a large number of those belonging to modern Western civilisation, the possibility of Lucifer and Ahriman taking hold of the matter of the brain becomes far greater. When however a human being begins 'to seek [and think about] the spiritual world in the form of materialism',[133] that is, by extending materialistic ideas directly to the occult realm, he becomes an 'occult materialist', and thereby creates particularly favourable conditions for strengthening the eighth sphere. Thus the constant growth of its forces in our time – as is shown in the form of physically visible phenomena – is the direct consequence of the general *materialistic character* of the modern era.

★

As we return to the theme of 'Shamballa' in Agni Yoga, it is necessary that we dwell at somewhat greater length upon its principal figure, who, according to Helena Roerich, unites both conceptions of Shamballa, its earthly and heavenly aspects. This figure is the Maitreya Bodhisattva. According to Helena Roerich's unshakeable conviction, the whole teaching ultimately derives from him.

Several times in her letters she also refers to her personal meeting with him, always calling him 'Gr.T.' (the great teacher): 'All the books of the teaching [Agni Yoga] bear witness to this direct contact. How could the experience of Agni

Yoga be arrived at without direct contact with the Gr[eat] T[eacher]? All the books, after all, were and are given by the Great Teacher on the basis of this experience [of clair-audience]'.[134] And in another letter this is spoken about still more concretely: 'I also saw the crystal of Materia Lucida [in Agni Yoga this is the primary element of matter lying at the foundation of the physically visible world], all this was shown to me by the Gr[eat] T[eacher]. Moreover, I was on two occasions on the verge of death by fire and was saved by the rays of the Gr[eat] T[eacher].'[135] Finally, at the very end of the fourth volume of *Agni Yoga*, Helena Roerich tells of her 'initiation' through the lord of Shamballa himself: 'Given in the valley of the Brahmaputra, which has its source in the lake of the Great Nagas, where the covenants of the Rig Veda are guarded*: "I laid the foundation of Agni Yoga on four ends like the pistil of a flower. I confirmed Agni Yoga with my steps and received the stone of fire into my hands. I gave the stone to her who in accordance with our resolve will be called the *Mother of Agni Yoga*" [henceforth the occult name of Helena Roerich].'[136]

As a result of this experience the image of the Maitreya gradually acquires truly cosmic dimensions in Helena Roerich's consciousness. He becomes the future ruler of the Earth, who unites in himself all the impulses of his predecessors and above all Buddha and Christ: 'The Great Spirit who stands at the head of the New Cycle will bear within himself the entire synthesis, all the greatest Manifestations of the past cycle. Hence the Synthesis of the Maitreya encompasses all Rays.'[137]

Regarding the Maitreya himself Helena Roerich says the

---

* The Roerichs visited the upper reaches of the Brahmaputra in April 1928, at the end of their great Himalayan expedition, on the way from Tibet to Sikkim (India).

following: 'It was also strange to read the words that "if the Lord Maitreya is to become a Buddha, He will probably come in a physical body". That individuality who according to the Eastern conception has the Aspect of the Maitreya became a Buddha long ago, that is, attained a high Enlightenment, with the result that the reason which you have adduced for physical incarnation falls away.'[138] And in another letter: 'The whole of the East believes in the coming of the L[ord] Maitreya, but those who know say that the L[ord] Maitreya now bears the form of the Lord of Shamballa and, of course, His Coming cannot be understood as a manifestation of His flesh amidst earthly conditions and earthly inhabitants.'[139]

These remarks are sharply at variance not only with classical Buddhist tradition but also with the spiritual-scientific research of Rudolf Steiner, according to which the Maitreya Bodhisattva, like his predecessor, the Bodhisattva Gautama, will incarnate on Earth again and again until after three thousand years he attains the stage of Buddhahood, when, as the first *Christian Buddha*, 'he will place everything at the service of the Christ impulse.'[140]

The activity of this new Bodhisattva can also be discerned in the 20th century. It is associated with the central spiritual event of our time, with the new appearance of Christ in the etheric body. For one of the fundamental truths of both esoteric and exoteric Christianity is the knowledge that after the fulfilment of the Mystery of Golgotha Christ will never return to the Earth in a physical body, just as He never appeared on Earth before His *sole* incarnation at the Turning-Point of Time in Jesus of Nazareth. To assert the contrary would signify a complete failure to understand either the Christ Being or the Mystery of Golgotha.

However, the new *supersensible* revelations of Christ, the consequence of His union with the whole of earthly evolution through the Mystery of Golgotha, will accompany and lead mankind throughout its future evolution. To begin with, these revelations will be etheric, then astral, and in the distant future at still higher levels.[141]

The first of these – Christ's manifestation in etheric form – has already begun in the 20th century and will gradually spread amongst mankind over the course of the next three millennia, during which time an ever greater number of people will quite naturally experience what the Apostle Paul experienced as a supersensible revelation of Christ on the road to Damascus.[142]

Proclaiming this to all humanity and preparing it for the new supersensible appearance of Christ is – in Rudolf Steiner's words – what the modern spiritual science, or Anthroposophy, founded by him is called upon to achieve: 'This great event, the new appearance of Christ [in etheric form], is manifested without books and documents for those who are worthily preparing for it. And it is the duty of Anthroposophy to proclaim this.'[143] For '. . . the movement of spiritual science exists for this reason. Its task is to create the conditions which make an understanding of the Christ possible on the physical plane, so that He may then be beheld [in supersensible form].'[144]

And if, on the one hand, the *whole* of Anthroposophy is to serve as a means of preparing humanity for this highly important event, the beginning of its proclamation – which Rudolf Steiner embarked upon in 1910 – was, on the other hand, accomplished by him out of the direct inspirations of the Maitreya Bodhisattva. He speaks about this in the tenth lecture of the lecture-cycle on the Gospel of St Matthew: 'And this Bodhisattva inspires us by making us aware that the time is approaching when the Christ will . . . appear as an enlivening force to men in a new form, in an *etheric* body.'[145]

From this same source of inspiration, Rudolf Steiner also reveals the true significance of the ancient Eastern teaching regarding the heavenly Shamballa. In his words, this is that ancient spirit-land which with the coming of Kali-Yuga and with the disappearance of the atavistic clairvoyance became invisible for earthly men but which will, from our time onwards, become accessible in a still greater majesty and glory to man's spirit-vision, appearing before him as that etheric sphere surrounding the Earth where the Etheric Christ can now be experienced: 'The appearance of Christ in His etheric form will be amongst the first things that human beings will perceive when Shamballa again becomes manifest. There is no one else who can lead mankind into the country which Oriental writings declare to have vanished other than the Christ. Christ will lead men to Shamballa ... Thus the new Christian confession will arise through our growing into that realm where we will first meet Him: through growing into the mysterious land of Shamballa.'[146]

This central spiritual reality of Shamballa – the living Christ, Who in His etheric body leads humanity into it and reveals Himself therein – was altogether unknown to the Roerichs. Their 'earthly Shamballa', lost somewhere in the inaccessible valleys of the Himalayas, has, in contrast, a wholly material character and is ruled by mahatmas for whom the mysteries of true Christianity are as yet beyond their reach. Hence the 'heavenly Shamballa', too, is for the Roerichs merely a repetition of ancient Shamballa, which in former times disappeared from human sight. The decisive metamorphosis through which it passed as a result of the Mystery of Golgotha, leading it to become in our time the spiritual sphere of activity of the Etheric Christ, was inaccessible and unknown both to the Roerichs and to the mahatmas who inspired them.

It follows from this that that other 'heavenly Shamballa', to which the Roerichs aspired, is none other than the realm of Lucifer – where Christ is not recognised – and his luciferic 'hierarchy of light'. For after the Mystery of Golgotha and Christ's union with the Earth, *everything* in earthly evolution that has not gained access to the sphere of Christ will inevitably sooner or later fall prey to Lucifer and Ahriman. It is in this sense that we should understand Helena Roerich's words that 'there is only one Hierarchy of Light, and this Hierarchy is of course the Trans-Himalayan Hierarchy',[147] that is, the hierarchy which serves Lucifer and, hence, knows nothing of either the true significance of the Mystery of Golgotha or the new etheric appearance of Christ.

Moreover, Helena Roerich's assertion – quoted above – that the Lord of Shamballa, the Maitreya, has already attained the stage of Buddhahood and will never appear on Earth again in a physical body but will only work in a spirit-body is very clearly an attempt to replace the Etheric Christ by that luciferic being whom she acknowledges as the Maitreya and as her, and her teaching's, inspirer.

Mention has already been made above (p. 12) of the endeavour on the part of the Eastern mahatmas to replace Christ with Lucifer. This falsehood has its source in one particular circumstance which Rudolf Steiner considers at some length in the lecture of 9 January 1912.[148] There he speaks of how the chief purpose and ultimate significance of the evolution of the present Earth is the full development by man of the *fourth* principle of his being, the principle of the ego. Thus Christ, in descending to the Earth, brought this central principle to mankind, though in its *macrocosmic* form, as the World Ego, which is the archetype of every human ego and at the same time its highest ideal. In contrast, the luciferic spirits will ever and again try to entice man towards the premature development of his higher principles: the Spirit-

Self, the Life-Spirit and even the Spirit-Man, that is, the fifth, sixth and seventh principles, though only in their *microcosmic* form. If the luciferic spirits succeed in obscuring the fundamental difference between macrocosmic and microcosmic evolution, they will be able to impress upon human beings the idea that the fifth, sixth and seventh principles are 'higher' than the fourth, which is to say that the false messiahs and teachers whom they possess are higher than the Christ.

The relationship of Agni Yoga to the luciferic realm as it has been characterised here is confirmed by one fact of interest, from which it is apparent that in the light of luciferic inspirations many truths can acquire a diametrically opposite meaning. Thus Helena Roerich transfers the dwelling place of the last guardian of the Grail, the mysterious Prester John or 'the sage of the great mountain', to 'earthly Shamballa', from where he sent news and messages to various earthly rulers, amongst whom was the conqueror, Genghis Khan: 'Thus Genghis Khan received advice from the Sage of the Great Mountain', writes Helena Roerich in one of her letters.[149] The fact that the direct inheritor of the impulses of Genghis Khan, his grandson Khan Batu, destroyed and burnt virtually the whole of Russia in 1238–40 and then subjected it to two hundred and fifty years of slavery, in all probability disturbed the Roerichs but little. After all, Nicholas Roerich dedicated a whole series of his pictures to Genghis Khan.

The reasons for this unusual sympathy for someone who was one of the cruellest conquerors in the entire history of humanity lie in the occult sphere. Thus in order to understand them it is necessary to turn to what has been given through modern spiritual science.

In the lecture of 17 September 1916[150] Rudolf Steiner indicated that it was Genghis Khan who in the 12th century received through a priestly emissary of a secret Mystery

Centre in the depths of Asia a *luciferic* initiation of unusual intensity and, associated with it, the task of 'gathering together everything that it was possible to gather from the forces of Asia and using this for the dissemination of what could lead the fifth post-Atlantean epoch back into a luciferic mould'. In other words, the mission of Genghis Khan was 'the great attempt – originating from Asia – to "visionise" [that is, give a visionary, atavistic character to] European culture and thereby cut it off from the conditions of further evolution, so as in a certain sense to draw it away from the Earth.'[151] Does not this aspect of the mission of Genghis Khan correspond to the underlying aspirations of the Roerichs in the 20th century?

The Roerichs also speak in this same spirit about the form of the Grail, which is for them merely a 'Great Stone in which magic powers are concentrated' and which has come from 'another planet'[152] or 'the chalice of Amrita',[153] the sacred drink of the East, with a similarity to soma. 'After all, the legend of the Grail Chalice came from the East and is one of the numerous accounts of that same Shamballa',[154] writes Helena Roerich in one of her letters; and in another letter she adds: 'Thus in its time it [the Chalice] was brought to the Lord Buddha . . . After the death of the Buddha, the Chalice was for a while in a Temple in Karashar, from whence it disappeared. Since this time it has been kept in Shamballa.'* [155]

There is no mention here of the connection of this chalice

* One of Helena Roerich's pupils, R. Rudsitis, the president of the Roerich Society in Riga in the thirties and forties, wrote a work by way of further development of these indications of hers under the title of 'Brotherhood of the Grail', in which he tried on the basis of historical and literary material to prove the Eastern Asiatic (Himalayan) origin of the whole cycle of legends of the Grail and even of the Arthurian knights. Extracts from it were recently printed in the journal of the Latvian Roerich Society, 'Uguns'.

with Christ. Hence the communion Chalice, hewn from the sacred stone, the 'Lapis Exillis', remains empty for the Roerichs, bereft of its true content – the blood of Christ. And this means that the stamp of Lucifer is also imprinted upon the Roerichs' 'Grail': this is an old chalice which has not become the Grail . . .

★

Another central idea of Agni Yoga – in addition to the teaching of the eternity of matter and the teaching of Shamballa – is that of fire. Hence its name: 'Yoga of Fire'. The fourth volume of the teaching bears this title, and its eighth, ninth and tenth volumes have the collective title of 'Fiery World'.

In a short definition of the principal terms of Agni Yoga, appended to a recent two-volume edition extracted from all fourteen volumes, we read: 'Agni Yoga is a yoga of fire. Fire is psychic energy'; 'The fiery world is a higher world of condensed light, the dwelling-place of higher souls.'★ It is in this sense that Helena Roerich writes in the eighth volume: 'The concept of Shamballa is inseparably connected with manifestations of fire'.[156]

In Agni Yoga the universe is divided into three levels: the 'world of density', corresponding to the physical plane; the 'refined world', which corresponds to the etheric and sometimes to the astral world; and the 'fiery world', corresponding to the mental or spiritual plane (the 'Devachan' of theosophy). The kindling of fire in the innermost heart is regarded by Agni Yoga as the entry into the sphere of cosmic fire, the fiery world. But here too the basic inadequacy of Agni Yoga becomes apparent: its total blindness to the sphere of Christ.

★ See the note on p. 70.

For since the Mystery of Golgotha the twofold mystery of fire in the cosmos and in man has been inseparably connected with the mystery of the Living Christ. Christ brought the true 'heavenly fire' to the Earth and, after passing through death and the Resurrection, appeared clothed in fire to the Apostle Paul on the road to Damascus: 'Christ appeared to Paul's enlightened gaze out of spiritualised fire'.[157] Henceforth 'Paul knew that Christ is alive when he saw Him manifested in spiritualised, blazing heavenly fire'.[158]

This central experience of Paul acquires a particular significance in our epoch of Christ's etheric revelation to mankind, which begins in the 20th century and will become increasingly widespread in the course of the next two and a half thousand to three thousand years. Hence Rudolf Steiner speaks of the 'Christians of the future': 'They will understand not only the Christ who passed through death but also the triumphant Christ of the Apocalypse, who resurrected in spiritual fire and whose coming has been foretold ... Thus the Christ is manifested ... in the spiritualised fire of the future. "He is with us always until the end of the world", and will appear in spiritual fire to those who allow their eyes to be illumined by the Event of Golgotha. Men will behold Him in spiritual fire. They will have first seen Him in another form, and only thereafter will they see the true form of Christ in spiritual fire.'[159]

This allusion to the general spiritualisation of the Earth, which began as a result of the Mystery of Golgotha through the spiritualising of the substance of fire (to be followed in future by the spiritualising of denser substances), is directly connected with the process whereby our Earth gradually becomes a new Sun, the radiant, fiery focus of the future cosmos. For now that He has as a result of the Mystery of Golgotha become the Spirit of the Earth, the Christ has kindled at its centre a new source of spiritual fire and spiritual light.[160]

But it is not only the macrocosmic mystery of 'heavenly fire' that is connected with the Event of Golgotha and the new etheric appearance of Christ. With them is also connected its microcosmic reflection in the human heart. For this organ is by no means merely what modern science considers it to be. From earliest times the mysterious process of the etherisation of earthly blood – a process which in occultism is also associated with fire – has been taking place in the human heart. The stream of this etherised blood flows from the heart to the head, and from thence out into man's spiritual environment. Thus one can say: the fire mystery which is continually being enacted in the human heart unites man with the higher supersensible world. However, this is not all there is to the fire mystery of the heart. For according to the testimony of modern spiritual research, since the Mystery of Golgotha another stream, that of the etherised blood of Christ, has flowed in every human being together with his own etherised blood from the heart to the head.[161]

In an ordinary human being these two etheric streams are not united, since in our time their union is inseparably connected with the assimilation of the true knowledge of Christ such as is given to modern man through Anthroposophy. But if such a union is achieved, it leads to a direct contemplation of the Etheric Christ in the spiritual world nearest to the Earth.[162] Thus the rightly understood and experienced microcosmic fire mystery, the mystery of the heart, leads man to an initiation into the macrocosmic fire mystery, to a contemplation in the macrocosm of Christ clothed in 'spiritualised heavenly fire', the source whereby the Earth will become in future a new Sun.

The fire mystery of the heart, in its old, pre-Christian form, is also spoken of – albeit in a very vague and confused way – in *Agni Yoga*, especially in the seventh volume, which is entitled 'The Heart'. However, Helena Roerich knows nothing about the mystery of the presence and influence in the human heart of the etherised blood of Christ, or the change that has come about in the relationship of the Earth and humanity to cosmic or heavenly fire as a result of the Mystery of Golgotha. Thus the fire that is spoken of in Helena Roerich's books is merely that primordial fire which – untouched by the transforming power of the Christ impulse – is in our time only capable of leading a human being who experiences it into the cosmic sphere of Lucifer, as is indicated in the central motif of the south green window in the First Goetheanum.

★

In Helena Roerich's books and letters, many additional examples can be found which testify to the complete inability of this occult stream to gain even a remote understanding of the truths of esoteric Christianity. Thus, for example, it is said of the present abode of Gautama Buddha that 'the Great Individuality of Buddha, His Fiery Ego, clothed with Materia Lucida [primal matter], dwells today in the spheres surrounding our planet'.[163] That the real Gautama Buddha, who has long been 'the most intimate pupil and friend of Christian Rosenkreutz',[164] was sent by him at the beginning of the 17th century to Mars, where he continues to abide even now for the fulfilment of a highly important spiritual mission, is something of which Helena Roerich – understandably enough – has no knowledge. Similarly, she regards Christian Rosenkreutz himself – this high initiate and leader of the whole stream of Christian esotericism – as merely one of the many teachers who tried to bring to Europe those same ancient teachings of the East, though outwardly endowing them with a 'semi-Christian aspect'. 'Thus, when Christian Rosenkreutz, the founder of the Rosicrucian Order, returned from Asia, he had to impart the Teaching of the East in a semi-Christian form, in order to defend his pupils from the persecution and vengeance of fanatics and hypocrites.'[165] Christian esotericism is viewed here merely as a protective cloak that has been cast over the treasures of Eastern knowledge for the purpose of diverting the attention of 'fanatics and hypocrites'.

Two further examples shall be cited, which have to do with temporal distortions in Agni Yoga. Thus the end of the dark age of Kali Yuga, which began in the year 3001 BC and ended – according to Rudolf Steiner's spiritual-scientific research – in 1899,[166] is postponed by Helena Roerich until 1942: '[Nineteen] forty-two is in all the ancient writings reckoned to be the end of Kali Yuga and the beginning of the new cycle of splendour.'[167] And in another letter she writes: 'The year [19]36 is denoted in all prophecies as the year of the beginning of the personal battle between the Arch[angel] Michael and the dragon'.[168] Whereas in Rudolf Steiner's spiritual-scientific research it is indicated that this battle began in 1841 and culminated in 1879 with Michael's victory and the beginning of the *modern epoch* of his rulership amongst mankind.[169]

★

In conclusion, a few words need to be said about the style in which the fourteen volumes of *Agni Yoga* are couched. Their principal feature is a strongly expressed poetic or mantric character, with numerous repetitions and variations of what is for the most part a simple selection of the same images and ideas, which with repeated reading over a long period – as is recommended – inevitably leads to one's waking, thinking consciousness being lulled to sleep. This effect is further intensified through the almost total absence in the text of concrete, cognitive elements or of the slightest aspiration towards a consistent logically ordered manner of exposition, such as the reader might be able to grasp with his individual cognitive faculties. The endless kaleidoscope of separate thoughts, incomplete images, frequently broken-off phrases, endless repetitions, the piling up of the same metaphors, and so on, eventually calls forth in the reader the feeling that he is in a surging and ceaselessly changing sea of images and rhythms, where any conscious control on the part of the individual ego is almost completely lost. And then the content can work in an unimpeded way upon the soul, like a hypnotic dream.

It is true that one can experience an inner world, a soul satisfaction, even bliss, but at the same time one is – imperceptibly – increasingly subject to the real danger of the uncontrollable influence of those forces and beings of whose nature one cannot gain the least idea from Agni Yoga. Thus it must be said that by excluding individual consciousness the content of Agni Yoga endeavours to exert a direct influence upon the deep, unconscious regions of the human soul, thus making man to a very high degree dependent upon this teaching and the mysterious mahatmas concealed behind it. In this sense its effect is comparable to a refined soul narcotic. And souls that have been prepared in this way are best able to serve as unconscious tools for the attainment of those goals which the Eastern mahatmas seek to reach with respect to the Slavic and especially the Russian peoples.

These goals, as is clear from what has been said hitherto, are associated with the endeavours of the [Asiatic] East to conquer true Christianity at any price and to replace it with ancient Tibeto-Indian wisdom, in order by this means to prevent the arising in the sixth post-Atlantean period of the universally human Christian culture which will be wholly founded on a new cosmic understanding of the Christ impulse, the establishing of which will be the task of the Russian people.

As was indicated at the beginning of this present work in the course of considering the first volume of *Agni Yoga* (see p. 18), its teaching is based on the absolute authority of the teacher. Helena Roerich emphasises this on several occasions in her letters: 'Yes, the Teaching of Living Ethics is based upon devotion to the Hierarchy of Light, upon a recognition of the high authority of the Teachers'.[170] From a practical point of view this increasingly leads modern man into a situation whereby he loses the most precious gift of earthly evolution, his free will, which can then be seized hold of by the opposing forces and drawn into the eighth sphere. For 'Lucifer and Ahriman are endeavouring to swallow man's free will up into the eighth sphere . . . And this means that man is continually subject to the danger that his free will is taken away from him and swallowed up in the eighth sphere.'[171]

Thus everyone who becomes acquainted with Agni Yoga should know that although it originates from a luciferic source it nevertheless – because of the blind adherence to the authority of teachers and the strong inclination towards the occult materialism developed under their influence – serves not only the aims of Lucifer but also of Ahriman, and that it is one of the very evident manifestations of their combined activity in the 20th century. This combination of forces can be withstood only by the true knowledge of the Mysteries of the Living Christ revealed in our time by Anthroposophy, which alone are capable of leading mankind into a future that is free from the forces of both Lucifer and Ahriman.

Postscript

After this study of the spiritual foundations of the occult stream founded by Helena and Nicholas Roerich had been completed, some material fell into the author's hands which rendered the following observations necessary.

The point at issue here is Helena Roerich's relationship to Anthroposophy and to its founder, Rudolf Steiner. Apart from a passing reference to the 'Steinerites' in one of her letters (HR II, 7 February 1936) – and, moreover, in a quotation – the writer of these lines has been unable to find any direct allusion to Anthroposophy amongst the writings of Helena and Nicholas Roerich to which he has had access. Of course, it is clear from all the facts adduced in the present work that there is a distinct antithesis between Anthroposophy, the representative of modern esoteric Christianity, and the teachings of Agni Yoga, which has its source in Indo-Tibetan occultism.

Such a general comparison would benefit from being made more concrete, from a final glance, as it were. This lack can now be remedied by the three-volume work by A. Kalizovsky, *Osnovy miroponimaniya novoi epokhi* ('Foundations of World Understanding in the New Epoch') republished in 1991 in Riga (in Russian), which represents a general exposition (almost 1000 pages) of the teachings of Agni Yoga, over half of which consists of quotations from its founder. Kalizovsky himself – a personal pupil of Helena Roerich – was in the thirties an executive member of the Latvian Roerich Society, and originally published his work in Riga in 1934 and dedicated it to his teacher. All three volumes, therefore, appeared during Helena Roerich's lifetime (she died in 1951).

Kalizovsky devoted the last six pages of the first volume to an analysis of Anthroposophy, and especially the personality of Rudolf Steiner, from the standpoint of Agni Yoga. Helena Roerich's opinion of Kalizovsky's book has also been preserved. But before giving the not merely positive but openly enthusiastic opinion of this book on the part of the founder of Agni Yoga, we shall cite here a few of its author's observations. It should be pointed out beforehand that in the following quotations Agni Yoga is completely identified with the second period of Helena Blavatsky's Theosophy, inasmuch as Helena Roerich regarded her teaching as a continuation of Blavatsky's mission in the 20th century.

Kalizovsky begins the section on Anthroposophy with the words: 'Apart from its overt and obvious enemies, Theosophy has others who are secret and, hence, more dangerous. Amongst these foes are Anthroposophy and its followers.' The reason for this is that 'shortly before Mrs Besant's death, the powers of darkness succeeded in recruiting Rudolf Steiner to the ranks of the Theosophical Society'. According to Kalizovsky, this happened in the following way: Rudolf Steiner 'reckoned that after Blavatsky's death he would be chosen as president of the Theosophical Society', whereas the mahatmas of the White Brotherhood chose not him but Annie Besant. 'As a result ... of this insult to his pride ... he abandoned Theosophy and founded Anthroposophy*', which was 'the

* The 'explanation' that Kalizovsky gives here as the reason for Rudolf Steiner's 'departure from Theosophy' is actually part and parcel of that slander which Annie Besant unleashed against Rudolf Steiner in the first decade of the century. In the lecture of 18 March 1916 (GA 174a) Rudolf Steiner called these fabrications of hers a 'conscious lie', inasmuch as in

first victory of the dark powers over Steiner'. For 'having gained mastery over such a capable colleague as Steiner, the dark powers gave their teaching [that is, Anthroposophy] to the world by using Steiner as their instrument'.

There then follows a thoroughly incompetent criticism of certain aspects of anthroposophical cosmology, a criticism which Kalizovsky does not base on the works of Rudolf Steiner himself – most likely he has never even read them – but, in his words, on 'a wholly objective judgement' which he has derived from a book written against Anthroposophy by a certain V. Goldenberg, *Antroposophskoye dvizhyeniye i yevo prorok* ('The Anthroposophical Movement and its Prophet').

However, all this is merely the prelude to addressing what is from the standpoint of Agni Yoga the principal 'error' of Anthroposophy and its founder. 'The Western world' – Kalizovsky continues – 'believes that Christ is the Only Son of the One God. *Steiner fully complies with this error*...' (italics S.P.). And then he goes on: 'People may say that it is hardly possible to regard Anthroposophy as a teaching of darkness when it has so high an estimation of Christ, when Anthroposophists are all zealous Christians and make efforts to combine Christianity with Anthroposophy. But the recognition of Christ by the powers of darkness is a generally known fact, for how could they fail to recognise Him? They have recognised Him post factum, but they have recognised Him in such a way as to shut out the possibility of recognising the next Teacher, for the formula that "One such as Christ

1909 he had personally and in the presence of witnesses '... clearly explained to her that ... [he] did not *under any circumstances* want to be more than the General Secretary of the German Section, or something along those lines'. (See also GA 167, lecture of 28 March 1916.)

there has never been and will never be again" shuts man off from all further progress, and this is all that is needed by the powers of darkness, it is for this reason that they recognise Him.'

It is evident from these words that it is precisely the principal result of Rudolf Steiner's spiritual-scientific research, with its testimony of the central significance of the Christ Being, as the Sun Logos, for our whole cosmos and of the Mystery of Golgotha for the whole of earthly evolution, which represents the main stumbling-block in Anthroposophy for the followers of Agni Yoga. For them, Christ is merely one of many teachers of mankind for whom they have equal reverence, merely the precursor of the 'next teacher' in the endless chain which Helena Roerich calls the 'Hierarchy of Light'. What she means by this she states in one of her letters: '. . . there is only one Hierarchy of Light, and this is the Trans-Himalayan Hierarchy' (HR II, 30 August 1935).

In Kalizovsky's opinion, Rudolf Steiner fell from this 'hierarchy': 'In calling Anthroposophy a teaching of the powers of darkness, the epithet of dark power must also be applied to the founder of this teaching. That this is neither calumny nor an insinuation is evident from the fact that Steiner rejected the heavenly Hierarchy that rules the world and did this wholly consciously, for Steiner – as a former theosophist – could not fail to know of its existence and that it rules the world. By rejecting the Hierarchy of Light, he thereby acknowledged the hierarchy of darkness.'

Yes indeed, by rejecting the hierarchy of the Indo-Tibetan mahatmas, which pursued only group and egotistically national interests, Rudolf Steiner was from the outset acknowledging only the true 'Heavenly Hierarchy' that serves the Cosmic Christ, of which Dionysius the Areopagite wrote out of the sources of esoteric Christianity. All the leading teachers of esoteric Christianity have always been directly associated with this true Heavenly Hierarchy, whose impulses they have endeavoured to bring to realisation amongst mankind, in the knowledge that 'Christ is the Ruler of *all* the beings of the higher Hierarchies' (GA 129, lecture of 21 August 1911).

As has been shown, the founder of Agni Yoga regarded Christ as a being who came – together with Gautama Buddha and the Maitreya Bodhisattva (in her opinion, the latter had long since attained the stage of Buddhahood, see p. 82) – from the planet Venus (see p. 70), that is, she saw in him a being who as regards his spiritual significance had not gone beyond the rank of Buddha. Her pupil Kalizovsky adds to this series of teachers 'Mohammed, Confucius' and, at one stroke, 'all the past and future Teachers of humanity'. In other words, according to the conception of Agni Yoga Christ is not a *Cosmic Being* Who lived *only once* on the Earth but merely one of many human initiates who, like them, has passed through many earthly incarnations before and since his life in Palestine at the beginning of the Christian era.

Once one has become familiar with this attitude of Agni Yoga to the Founder of Christianity, it is not difficult to distinguish the true sources of such ideas. In his descriptions in his lectures of how the luciferic and ahrimanic powers battle against the Christ impulse (which is to say, against the true evolution of humanity), Rudolf Steiner often spoke of the way in which Lucifer tries to represent Christ's earthly life in Palestine as a kind of illusion or beautiful legend, whereas Ahriman endeavours to portray Christ merely as one of many earthly initiates, as a being who does indeed stand at a higher level in his development than 'Socrates or Plato' but who nonetheless belongs wholly to the human race.

But this conception of Christ, according to which His

higher cosmic, divine Nature completely disappears and only the human, earthly aspect remains, is not simply a special form of modern materialism (cf. p. 44) but is, in Rudolf Steiner's words, one of the most effective means whereby Ahriman is in our time preparing for his future incarnation amongst mankind, in order – by appearing on Earth as a new and higher teacher – to attempt to lead earthly evolution in the direction that he desires.*

Kalizovsky's criticism of Anthroposophy springs ultimately from these overtly ahrimanic influences – which are also the source of its manifest coarseness. Not mincing his words, over the course of barely six pages he calls Anthroposophy a 'human fabrication', the 'ravings of a disordered imagination', 'a cunningly conceived net to catch people in', 'a great deception', 'tares which the enemy of humanity has sown amongst the wheat', and so on.

Finally, drawing upon 'information from highly authoritative sources', Kalizovsky asserts that the influence of the 'powers of darkness' was most strongly manifest in the last six years of Rudolf Steiner's life. In the context of Kalizovsky's treatise, this 'highly authoritative source' can only be the founder of Agni Yoga, Helena Roerich, together with Nicholas Roerich or the Himalayan mahatmas standing behind them, and quite possibly both the former and the latter together. Now the last six years of Rudolf Steiner's life were the time when he embarked upon the revelation in all their depth of the Michael Mysteries of our cosmos. Precisely from

* Rudolf Steiner tells of Ahriman's incarnation on Earth, which is to come about at the beginning of the third millennium, and about the preparation for this incarnation in our time in the lectures published in GA 191 and GA 193. There it is indicated that this incarnation will take place in the American West.

this period (1919–25)*, his relationship with the high sphere of the Time-Spirit, Michael, acquired such a concrete and intense character that it can be said in full accord with the occult reality that through Rudolf Steiner, the modern Christian initiate, Michael, the cosmic 'Countenance of Christ', was active to an ever greater degree from this time onwards, and through his greatest pupil founded on Earth the New Christian Mysteries, whose task it is to serve the true Heavenly Hierarchy led in the spiritual world by Christ Himself.†

And as from Ahriman's point of view everything coming from the sphere of Michael is seen as darkness, in that he is spiritually blind to its influences, it is completely clear that this activity of Michael as expressed through Rudolf Steiner must be perceived by Ahriman as 'darkness' or as a 'power of darkness'.

This also sheds light upon the real inspirer of those 'highly authoritative sources' upon which Kalizovsky and his guru, Helena Roerich, drew in their spiritual blindness. Thus Helena Roerich writes to him in a letter from India after she became acquainted with the text of the work whence all the remarks about Anthroposophy and its founder quoted above are taken: 'Your excellent work has brought great joy. This is what is so urgently necessary now, for we must do all we can to stir the awareness that has been buried in musty prejudices

---

* This period begins with the lecture-cycle 'The Mission of the Archangel Michael, the Revelation of the Essential Secrets of Man's Being' (November 1919, GA 194), and ends with the articles on 'The Michael Mystery' (August 1924–March 1925, GA 26).

† For further details regarding the last years of Rudolf Steiner's life and his relationship to the sphere of Michael in this period, see S.O. Prokofieff, *Rudolf Steiner and the Founding of the New Mysteries*, Rudolf Steiner Press 1986.

and crushed by the horrors of this terrible age. The light of the new era is dawning, and we must be able to meet it with an awake spirit. I await with impatience the continuation of your work, which should be printed and widely disseminated. Your work, which so clearly sets forth the problems of Existence, is of the greatest value, and we hope that you will continue in this direction. The Teaching of Life contains so many new themes which have not as yet been touched upon!'*

★

In conclusion, it should be pointed out that the stream of Agni Yoga, despite its rapid spread in recent times in a number of the countries of Europe, America and, in particular, Eastern Europe (Russia, Latvia and so on), would not perhaps have merited such great attention if it had not been connected in a quite special way with another occult stream, which has achieved a wide dissemination above all in the West, namely the movement founded by the Englishwoman Alice Bailey and generally known under the name 'Servants of the World' or the 'Secret School' (Schola arcana).

The fact of the matter is that both these movements derive from one and the same occult centre, whose leaders sent the Russian, Helena Roerich, to the East so as to spread their teachings from India via Tibet and Mongolia to Russia, and – at almost exactly the same time – the Englishwoman, Alice Bailey, to the West, for the attainment of the same aims via America. (The occult stream of Alice Bailey will be considered in the second part of the present work, which will be published separately.)

---

* This quotation is cited in the publisher's foreword to the first volume of Kalizovsky's work.

If we now view both streams as two mutually complementary parts of *one* all-embracing plan, we shall be able to sense the true extent of the very real spiritual battle which is being waged in the 20th century behind the scenes of outer events against the very *meaning of the Earth*, which consists in 'knowledge, and fulfilment of the intentions, of the *Living Christ*' (Rudolf Steiner).

And if it is the task of Anthroposophy today to help towards the immediate fulfilment of these higher intentions, the first step in this direction must be to *understand* as clearly and as deeply as possible the whole meaning and true significance of the battle being waged here, in which all anthroposophists are also involved. It has been the main purpose of the present book to contribute towards the development of such a deeper understanding.

Supplement I. The Roerichs and the Gorbachevs (see p. 1)

The friendly relations between the Gorbachevs and the last representative of the Roerichs' family are not fortuitous. For in one particular area their opinions strongly coincide. This concerns the relationship of both M. Gorbachev and S. Roerich to the mission of Lenin, the events of 1917 and the subsequent 75 years of Bolshivik rule in Russia (see also the Appendix).

That Gorbachev has not altered his convictions on this matter – convictions which he has previously expressed more than once as General Secretary and as President – now that he has for some time been merely a private individual is apparent from his last interview, given to the German newspaper *Der Spiegel*. This interview was published in January this year (issue no. 3, 1993) and gives further confirmation of the fact that, from the very beginning of *perestroika*, Gorbachev did not want to abolish but merely to reform Bolshevik socialism in Russia, by restoring it to its sources – that is, to its original Leninist principles, to which Gorbachev, like S. Roerich and his parents, remained faithful to the end. We shall cite here some extracts from this interview.

Der Spiegel: 'For three generations Russia was a field of experiment for state socialism. Why Russia: historical accident, or was there a national predisposition for this?'

Gorbachev: 'We should not become mystical about it, but set 1917 in its real context. And then we must ask ourselves what was wrong . . . and why it was with us . . . that the Bolsheviks came to power? Because the alternative was military dicatatorship.'

This completely mythical justification for the Bolsheviks coming to power has been reiterated by Gorbachev also while he was General Secretary and President of the USSR, seemingly forgetting that from 1917 onwards the Bolsheviks established in Russia a dictatorship which in its cruelty and criminality surpassed all dictatorial regimes that have ever existed in the history of mankind.

Later in the interview, when asked about the past 75 years of Bolshevik rule, Gorbachev replied: 'I would not wish to dismiss these seven and a half decades as a period when nothing positive or democratic occurred, when there was no freedom or social justice . . .'

The German correspondent, doubtless astonished at such a candid remark, could not restrain himself from asking a direct question: 'Can it be that you are still a communist?' Gorbachev's answer is somewhat evasive, but sufficiently clear in its meaning: 'I shall simply say that there are things which should not be forgotten and which the people do not wish to renounce'.

One might well suppose that these words would be completely subscribed to by not only all the members of the Roerich family but also by their Himalayan inspirers.

Supplement II. The Eastern Mahatmas and the Western World (see p. 8)

Rudolf Steiner speaks as follows about Blavatsky's liberation from her occult prison by Indian occultists: 'Certain Indian occultists now came to know of the affair [that Blavatsky had become occultly imprisoned], occultists who on their part tended strongly to the left [which in occult terminology means those who belonged to the "left", egotistical path], and whose prime interest it was to direct the occultism which was to be given to the world through H. P. Blavatsky in such a way that it could influence the world in line with the specific interests of Indian occultists' (GA 254, lecture of 11 October 1915).

The potential for this change from the universally human interests displayed in *Isis Unveiled* to the specific interests of the 'Tibeto-Indian' mahatmas, which were manifested with particular intensity in her chief work, *The Secret Doctrine*, had its deeper roots in the karmic guilt of the West for the 'innumerable injustices' which it had perpetrated over the centuries on the Asiatic East. Rudolf Steiner says in this connection: 'India, whose occult endeavours had been suppressed, took karmic revenge by impregnating the first manifestation of occultism in the West with its own egotistic, national occultism. This took place in the time of H. P. Blavatsky ... Her first work, *Isis Unveiled*, shows her to be a person of a thoroughly chaotic, illogical, passionate and confused nature, but it also shows that behind her there stand vigilant powers [associated with true Rosicrucianism, see Supplement VII], which seek to direct her towards universally human concerns. In *The Secret Doctrine* – quite apart from its very evident stature – everything is dominated by narrowly human interests, interests stemming from certain occult centres which in our time do not concern themselves with affairs of a universally human nature but only with a certain specific aspect. Both the Tibeto-Indian and the Egyptian initiation* of modern times always only have specific, limited interests in view; they want to avenge themselves upon the Western world for having suppressed Eastern occultism, for having overwhelmed the world of the East with materialistic influences' (address to Russian members, 11 April 1912, GA 158). The 'certain occult centres' referred to here are the chief centre of the mahatmas in the Himalayas and the monasteries and ashrams connected with it; and the 'Tibeto-Indian initiation' is the principal source of *The Secret Doctrine* and of theosophical teaching as a whole (in the second phase of its development), a teaching which, in the words of the most well-known Russian biographer of Blavatsky, E. Pisareva (see Supplement III), 'expresses the views of certain groups of *Tibetan Buddhists*' to which Blavatsky added 'the idea of evolution and perfection, and also an explanation of the origin of the universe ... which was adopted from brahmanism'.†

It is interesting that in one of the lesser-known works of Blavatsky it is possible to find unexpected confirmation that these group-egotistical and even politically tinged aims of the Himalayan mahatmas indeed existed. Thus in her book *From*

* In the fourteenth volume of *Agni Yoga*, the mahatma dictating to Helena Roerich says that 'the last Egyptian ashram had to move to the Himalayas', section 19 (*AY*).

† E. Pisareva, 'The Mission of Blavatsky, Theosophy and the Theosophical Society', published in a collection entitled *Aum*, New York and Moscow 1989.

the Caves and Jungles of Hindustan, which consists of travel notes written by Blavatsky for a Russian journal in the 1880s, she gives a detailed description of her meetings and conversations with one of the mahatmas, who accompanied her and her companions during part of the journey in India. In the book he is presented under the name of Gulab Lall Singh, behind which identity is concealed the mahatma Morya; despite the fact that in the letters to Sinnett the mahatma Kut Humi was also often referred to under the name of Lall Singh (see Helena Roerich's comments about this in her letters of 14 August 1936 *HR II*). However, there is something else which is of importance here. In a conversation with an American, a member of the expedition, whom she calls 'Colonel O.' (presumably Olcott), Blavatsky says of Morya-Lall Singh: 'I know him better than you ... Let us thank destiny that he, who sees better than any other that we – despite belonging to the "white race" which he hates and despises – are ardently devoted to him and, perhaps even more important, have a sincere sympathy for his people and a respect for his country, makes for us a unique exception [accepts two 'whites' as his occult pupils]. Do not demand of him what he cannot and will be unable to give us, and be content with the crumbs [of wisdom] which he throws to us on the road.'*

These words about the 'white race' which the mahatma 'hates and despises' (by which is meant Euro-American humanity) fully correspond in their meaning and especially in their emotional mood to Rudolf Steiner's remark quoted above about the efforts of Tibeto-Indian initiates to take vengeance upon the Western world on behalf of suppressed Eastern occultism.

* H.P. Blavatsky, *From the Caves and Jungles of Hindustan*, ch. xxix, London 1892.

Supplement III. H.P. Blavatsky and the Eastern Mahatmas (see p. 8)

The following words of E.F. Pisareva, Blavatsky's follower and biographer, active theosophist and translator into Russian of many theosophical works, describe *from theosophical sources* the history of Blavatsky's selection by the mahatmas as the mediator between them and Western humanity*: 'This question [regarding the spread of Eastern occult teachings to the West] was discussed in the lamaist monastery of Halaring Sho near Shigatse, which is on the border between China and Tibet.† The people who resolved this question were philosopher-ascetics with a deeply meditative life, who in the hierarchy of humanity stand far higher than us . . .' However, most of the participants – according to Pisareva – did not support this idea and only two of those who were present were in favour of it happening. 'These were the voices of two Hindus: Morya, a descendant of the rulers of Punjab, and Kut Humi, who came from Kashmir. They took upon themselves

---

* E.F. Pisareva, 'The Mission of H.P. Blavatsky, Theosophy and the Theosophical Society', article in the collection entitled *Aum*, New York–Moscow 1991. In a note to her letter of 23 October 1936 (vol. II), Helena Roerich makes special mention of Pisareva's biography of Blavatsky.

† Subsequently, the Roerichs visited these places during their Himalayan expedition. In the book *Heart of Asia*, published in New York in 1930, Nicholas Roerich – without, it is true, mentioning the monastery of Halaring Sho – writes: 'Near the region of Shigatse, on the picturesque banks of the Brahmaputra, . . . there still were until quite recently ashrams of the Himalayan Mahatmas'.

the responsibility for choosing the emissary and directing her to the West, in order that she might disseminate there *the philosophy of Brahmanism* and reveal a portion of the secrets concerning the nature of man ... And the choice fell upon H.P. Blavatsky... Why was she chosen and not someone endowed with a more even temper, the power to convince, disciplined intellectual capacities and an absence of passion – qualities which H.P. Blavatsky has always lacked?' Pisareva herself gives the following answer to this question: 'She [Blavatsky] was chosen because of her unusual mediumistic gifts and her paranormal faculties, which she had had since childhood. These faculties enabled her teachers, Morya and Kut Humi, to communicate easily with her at a distance by means of telepathy, that is, to impart higher knowledge to her by means of mediumistic dictation and astral demonstration, which played an important part in the writing of her *Secret Doctrine* and in the origin of the so-called 'letters of the mahatmas'. For the same reason, Blavatsky said on more than one occasion to her sister, V. Zhelikhovskaya, that she would never have arrived at the ideas contained in her works 'with her mind'.*

* Extracts from Zhelikhovskaya's memories of her conversations with Blavatsky are to be found in the journal, '*Nauka i religiya* ('Science and Religion') No. 9, 1991.

Supplement IV. The Visit by Tibetans to Russia (see p. 27)

The attempts of certain Tibetans to enter Russia and gain influence over its policy with regard to Asia and Europe are attested by the following facts.

In the last third of the 19th century two brothers of Buryat origin came to St Petersburg from Tibet. They were direct descendants of Genghis Khan; one of them was a lama, and the other was a doctor, a specialist in Tibetan medicine. The russified name of the latter was Pyotr Badmayev. In St Petersburg the brothers established the first Tibetan pharmacy and opened a medical practice. Between 1875 and 1892 P. Badmayev had almost a quarter of a million patients, which led to the tsar, Alexander III, granting him the title of Privy Councillor.

Having thus developed a connection with the Petersburg court, Badmayev soon submitted a written proposal to the tsar for a plan for a bloodless union of the Russian Empire with China, Mongolia and Tibet, merely requesting the necessary material support for this – to begin with, the two million gold roubles by means of which, for the fulfilment of his intentions, Badmayev proceeded to found the Russo-Asiatic firm of P.A. Badmayev and Co. The plan itself was as follows: to profit from the discontent with the ruling Manchurian dynasty that was at the time widespread amongst the Chinese people and, with the help of clever propaganda and bribery and if necessary with the support of a small contingent of the Russian army, 'to capture the strategic point [the town of

Lan-chou-fu] without bloodshed. [For] from this point it is very simple to extend influence throughout China, Tibet and Mongolia' (from Badmayev's memorandum to Tsar Alexander III of 13 February 1893 entitled 'The Tasks of Russia in the Asiatic East').

The Minister of Finance, Witte,* who initially supported Badmayev's plan, wrote to Alexander III as follows about the Badmayev project: 'The whole undertaking, as said, must have a completely private character and be conducted in an entirely unofficial way, with no more than material support' (memorandum of 27 February 1893). And he continues in the same vein: 'If the enterprise yields the results expected by Mr Badmayev, Russia – from the shores of the Pacific Ocean and the heights of the Himalayas – will hold sway not only in Asiatic but also in European affairs.'

However, it appeared that there was not enough money for the fulfilment of Badmayev's plan, and so after a certain time he again turned to the tsar for financial help, this time to Nicholas II, who in the meantime had ascended the throne. In a letter of 19 December 1896 Badmayev, endeavouring in every way he could to convince the tsar of the political advantages of his enterprise, wrote to him: '... my activities have the aim that Russia should have greater influence than other powers upon the Mongolian-Tibetan-Chinese East'. Badmayev made particular efforts to oppose the English in the East. In connection with this he even sent the tsar a special memorandum entitled 'On Opposing the English in Tibet', where he wrote, in particular: 'Tibet, which – as the highest plateau of Asia – rules over the Asiatic continent, must without doubt be in the hands of Russia. By commanding this

* Subsequently, on the eve of the First World War, Witte came out against Badmayev's plans.

point, Russia will surely be able to make England more compliant'.

Nevertheless, the enterprise soon folded up, since Badmayev was unable to obtain money from Nicholas II for the further implementation of his project. It is not impossible that a significant part was played in this by Rasputin, who did all he could to oppose the influence of the Tibetans on the tsar.

Badmayev saw the principal guarantee for the success of his enterprise in the wide diffusion in Mongolia, China and Tibet of the legends about the 'white tsar' who was to come from the North (from 'Northern Shamballa') and restore the violated and now decadent traditions of true Buddhism. In his memorandum to Alexander III quoted above ('The Tasks of Russia in the Asiatic East'), he cites some of these legends. One of these is of particular interest, and in the memorandum there is the following observation about it: 'In the seventh century after the death of Genghis Khan, who died in 1227, a white standard is expected to appear in Mongolia from Russia'.

If we add 700 years to 1227 we arrive at 1927, at the beginning of which the trans-Himalayan expedition under Roerich's leadership, which had left Moscow under the tanka (banner) of Shamballa, finally reached the Mongolian capital, Ulan-Bator. Here Helena Roerich published the third volume of *Agni Yoga*, *Community*, with all its adulations of Lenin and Bolshevik ideology by the Himalayan mahatmas, and also the book *The Foundations of Buddhism* (see Appendix). If we now recall that Nicholas Roerich said that he went to Mongolia in order to fulfil certain 'assignments on behalf of the mahatmas' (*EP**), we have here a definite connection between the activities of Badmayev and the Roerichs, behind

* See list of abbreviations on p. 159.

whom in both cases there stood one and the same impulse of the Himalayan occultists.

Finally, Roerich's great plan of 'uniting Russia and the vast world of Buddhism with the help of the mahatmas' (*EP*), which – at the behest of the latter – he explained at some length in a conversation with the People's Commissar for Foreign Affairs, Chicherin, in 1926 in Moscow and regarding which – albeit in different words – H. Roerich wrote in her letters to President Roosevelt, can in all essentials be found in Badmayev's letters to the Russian tsars.

This same tendency can be discerned in Blavatsky, inasmuch as in the last period of her life she was under the ever growing influence of the Tibeto-Indian occultists. Rudolf Steiner says in this connection: 'But one of these factors [that influenced Blavatsky] was the endeavour to join India to Asia [that is, Mongolia, Tibet and China], in order with the help of the Russian Empire to create an Asiatic-Indian dominion. And so these teachings [of Blavatsky] took on an Indian aspect, in order that in this way the West might be conquered. As you may see, this represents the incursion of a one-sidedly egotistic, nationalistic element' (GA 258, lecture of 14 June 1923). And the three-year trans-Himalayan expedition of the Roerichs, with its culmination of the visit to Moscow, was also to serve the same purpose.

But let us return to Badmayev. In St Petersburg he had an association with a highly placed Tibetan, the lama Agvan Dordzhiyev (1854–1938), the tutor and principal confidant of the 13th Dalai Lama. With the blessing of the latter he opened the first Buddhist temple on the territory of European Russia, the construction of which was at that time supported by N. Roerich. He was even included by Dordzhiyev in his construction committee. The temple was dedicated to 'Kalachakra', a Tibetan teaching about which Roerich's elder son,

Yuri, later wrote a treatise. Subsequently, in the 1950s, on returning to Russia, Yuri belonged to a group of people who were actively promoting the revival of the temple.

Probably before the beginning of the First World War, an even more significant figure of the Tibetan world, the lama Lubsan Sandal Tsydenov (born 1842), who bore the very rare title of 'Dharma Radzhi' ('tsar of learning'), visited St Petersburg at the head of a Buryat delegation through the mediation of lama Dordzhiyev. It could be supposed that the negotiations were most likely conducted along the same lines as those of Badmayev. However, they did not lead to any perceptible success, as the following episode – in particular – makes manifest. During the official reception at the Winter Palace, when Nicholas II entered the reception-room where the Buryat delegation was waiting with Tsydenov at its head and all those present immediately knelt according to etiquette, the 'tsar of learning' alone remained standing. His answer when asked about such incivility was: 'A spiritual tsar does not bow down before a worldly tsar'.

As a result the Buryat delegation had to pay a substantial penalty, and nothing further is known about the subsequent negotiations. On the eve of the Bolshevik Revolution it was probably decided in the occult circles of Tibet to achieve the aims referred to above not through the 'white' but through the 'red tsar', as is attested by the fact of the mahatmas' timely visit to Lenin in Switzerland (see p. 26) and also their message sent in 1926 through N. Roerich to the Bolshevik government (see p. 37f.).*

---

* The following sources were used for the writing of this appendix: *Za kulissami tsarizma* (Archiv tibetskovo vracha Badmayeva) ('Behind the Scenes of Tsarism' (the archive of the Tibetan doctor, Badmayev)), published in Russia in 1925, the article in the journal *Nauka i religiya*

In conclusion, it should also be pointed out that what is said here does not relate to the traditional Eastern religions as such but only to the so-called streams of the 'left wing', which concern themselves with occult politics and strive towards the spiritual conquest of the Christian West (see Supplement VIII).

('Science and Religion') about Agvan Dordzhiyev of 2 February 1990, the foreword to Badmayev's handbook on Tibetan medicine recently republished in Moscow and A.I. Andreyev's brochure, *Buddhiskaya svyatynya Petrograda* ('The Buddhist sanctuary of Petrograd').

Supplement V. The Roerichs and Franklin D. Roosevelt (see p. 31)

The correspondence which H. Roerich conducted with the American President F.D. Roosevelt in the period between October 1934 and January 1936 acquires a particular significance in this connection. Nine of these letters to the president were recently published in Moscow in translation from English (the originals are kept in the Franklin D. Roosevelt Library in New York).* Despite their pathetic style and thoroughly muddled content, the large number of vague allusions and areas of incomprehensibility, one aspect at any rate presents itself in them with sufficient clarity. (From the beginning of Helena Roerich's letter, it is apparent that there must have been answering 'messages' on the part of the president though it is not clear whether they were written or merely in verbal form through intermediaries. It was when this correspondence was in full swing that Roosevelt signed the cultural pact of N. Roerich in the White House on 15 April 1935, a deed which was doubtlessly the expression of the influence of these letters.)

Already in the first and longest of the letters (dated 10 October 1934), which was written shortly after the Roerichs' return from America to India, to the Kulu valley, there is a very clear indication that these letters were written at the

---

* In the annual publication, *Mir cherez kulturu* ('Peace through culture'), published by Sovyetsky Pisatyel, Moscow 1990. [The present renderings have been made from the Russian translation – Translator's note.]

behest, and at times according to the direct dictation (these parts of the letters are in inverted commas in the original), of the mahatmas standing behind Helena Roerich.

The first letter begins thus: 'Mr President, at this weighty hour, when the whole world stands at the threshold of reconstruction and the destinies of many countries hang in the Cosmic Balance, I write to you from the heights of the Himalayas in order to offer you Help from Above: Help from that Source which since times immemorial has been ceaselessly on the alert, observing the course of world events and directing it along paths of salvation'. And the letter goes on to enumerate a whole series of examples, where mysterious individuals have been sent by the Himalayan brotherhood to Europe and America in order to exert an influence upon the historical destiny of mankind. Thus the 'first Habsburg' was visited by a certain knight-troubadour; the Norwegian King Knut by an unknown figure in a pilgrim's garb; and Marie Antoinette by the Count of St Germain, who was, according to Roerich, also 'a member of the Himalayan brotherhood'.

Then the letter mentions some warnings given by certain mysterious individuals to Napoleon, Queen Victoria and the Swedish King Charles XII; reference is made to a 'grave warning' which was given from the same source to the government of Russia and to the 'sad consequences of its being ignored' and so on. Then it speaks of the advice which was given to George Washington by an anonymous professor; and of the decisive appearance of a mysterious stranger when America adopted the declaration of independence, and so forth. And this lengthy catalogue ends with the words: 'Thus in the course of history it is possible to be a witness of the various ways in which Help, Warnings and Advice from higher sources have been manifested. And this advice issuing from the Great Source was always easy to carry out and has never harmed the country for which it was intended'. Today 'Advice has been made ready for America, and it would be well to accept it, for there are many examples of the sad consequences of rejection'. After this long introduction Helena Roerich now turns directly to the president himself: 'You can be not only a Ruler but a truly great Leader. From now on the Mighty Hand extends Help to you from this One Source and the Fiery Messages can again reach the White House'.

In the next letter, of 15 November 1934, Helena Roerich writes: 'My heart has joy in transmitting the following Great Words to you: "Despite the opposition the Country has not known a better loved President. His fame will grow. That is predestined."' And then she continues: 'And now I shall quote verbatim the indications that I have received...'

The following picture gradually emerges from this and subsequent letters of the nature of the secret intentions of the 'One Source' standing behind Helena Roerich, a picture which consists of certain elements:

(a) 'The country [the USA] should not disarm but, on the contrary, its power shall make itself felt. And although the nation may be against armaments, one should not defer to this, since no one will dare to attack a powerful ruler' (letter of 15.11.1934). And in another letter (of 27.12.1935): 'America must stand as a power that is mightily armed and equipped'.

(b) 'All Cosmic conditions are favourable to the secret negotiations of the President, negotiations which should not be divulged by the press nor by those surrounding him. The President must therefore work through those who are devoted to him and are sincerely disposed towards him. Thus we look towards the establishing of a Union, which will in future unite S[outh] A[merica] with the USA and Pr[esident Roosevelt] will become the founder of this Great State. This

Great Union is already determined and will come about' (letter of 27.12.1934). Then in the same letter Helena Roerich again turns to the president: 'May the Pr[esident] be the Great Uniter of this mighty Country, which is destined to play a Great part in the Cosmic Balance. This vital question will be resolved, and Help will be granted to the Pr[esident].'

(c) 'But the President's attention must be turned towards the East. In speaking of the East, We also mean Russia ... A Great State is arising in the East. This new beginning will bring that equilibrium which is so urgently necessary for the building of the great Future ... And so the time has come for the reconstruction of the East and may there be friends of the East in America. The union of the peoples of Asia is something that has been decided, the union of the tribes and peoples will gradually come about, it will be something akin to a Federation of countries. Mongolia, China and the Kalmuks will form a counterweight to Japan, and for this union of peoples Your Good Will is necessary, Mr President'(letter of 4 February 1935). This 'good will' of the president was in particular, in the opinion of the mahatmas standing behind Helena Roerich, to serve to 'save [from hunger] the needy of China' (letter of 15 April 1935).

From the sections that have been quoted there is evidence of a need for the maximum possible military strengthening of North America and the subjection of South America to its power. Thus united, America was – in the minds of the mahatmas – to represent a Western world bloc. On the other hand, an Eastern world bloc – consisting of Russia, China, Mongolia and the Kalmuks (including Tibet – see supplement IV) – was also to arise.

The relationships between these two world blocs are then characterised in a thoroughly contradictory way. On the one hand, 'so-called Russia will be a counterbalance to America, and only through such an order will the problem of World Peace be solved' (letter of 4 February 1935). And on the other hand, we read in the same letter: 'America has already long been connected with Asia. The old connections were strengthened under favourable configurations of the Stars. What has been foreordained by Cosmic Laws will inevitably be accomplished. To no one is it given to hamper or block the path of the Enlightened Ones. Consequently, everyone must acknowledge the truth that the peoples who occupy the greater part of Asia are destined to respond to America's friendship. The President can receive the counsel of happiness. May the President's powers be employed in consolidating the situation. The President can at the designated hour direct his peoples with a firm hand towards the Union which will establish equilibrium in the World. One may employ small-scale measures, but must aspire to greater things. We send this message which can strengthen the President's will and bring it into accordance with the rays of the Enlightened Ones.' This is reminiscent of Nicholas Roerich's words from his book *Heart of Asia*: 'The heights of Asia and the heights of America will reach out their hands to one another...'*

And at the end of her message Helena Roerich communicates to the president the following words of the mahatmas standing behind her: 'Our Ray is over President Roosevelt. A new dawn rises over America' (letter of 4 February 1935), and from herself personally she sends him 'an ancient symbolic image of the Lord of Shamballa', with the request that he accept this 'Image which is sacred to me [H. Roerich] and remember that the Ray of the Great God will accompany You...'.

---

* The book was published in New York in 1930.

Despite the confused and contradictory nature of what is expressed, there nevertheless emerges from the letters – as has been said – a pretty clear picture of the opposition, and at the same time the common ground (perhaps first the one and then the other), between the Western and Eastern worlds. The result and ultimate goal of such a constellation – although of course this is not spoken of directly in the letters – must be *the exclusion of the creative middle, expressed by Christian Europe*, from human evolution and the establishing of an at times mutually antagonistic and at times mutually unifying *world dualism*, in the sense of the fundamental principal of Agni Yoga: the uniting of the materialistic West with the ancient, pre-Christian spirituality of the East, which on an occult plane signifies the realisation of a synthesis – embracing the entire planet – of ahrimanic and luciferic forces with, if possible, the total exclusion of the Christian impulse of the middle (cf. Supplement VII).

Already in 1919 Rudolf Steiner called this dualistic principle – wherever it appears – 'the delusion or madness of dualism', and explained its nature as follows: 'Everything that works within this delusion is essentially the result of ahrimanic influences, of those influences which will come to a focus in the incarnation of Ahriman, of which I have often spoken [in other lectures]' (GA 194, 21 November 1919).*

The only thing that can withstand this is a true esoteric knowledge of the cosmic significance of the Christ impulse, as has now been given to humanity in Anthroposophy. For only through attaining a completely new and fully conscious relationship to the Christ impulse is it possible to establish a real balance in the world between the luciferic and ahrimanic

* Regarding the future incarnation of Ahriman in the American West, see the Postscript.

forces and thus furnish humanity with the opportunity for further evolution on Earth. 'On the scales of world existence we have the luciferic element, representing the one arm, and the ahrimanic element, representing the other arm, while the Christ-impulse represents the state of equilibrium.' (ibid.)

Supplement VI. Jesus 'in India'
(see p. 33)

The persistence and consistency displayed by Roerich in his quest for the secret manuscript which confirmed the 'fact' of Jesus Christ's stay in India and Tibet are apparent from the following notes written in his own hand in the diary that he kept of his journey*: 'The existence of manuscripts about Jesus is at first completely denied. Of course the denial springs primarily from missionary circles. Then, by degrees, fragmentary and tentative information gradually emerges which is arrived at only with great difficulty. Finally, it transpires that some old people in Ladakh (Northern Kashmir) have heard of and know the manuscripts. Such documents as the manuscripts about Christ and the book about Shamballa lie in a very "dark" [secret] place.'

'Three pieces of information in one day about a manuscript concerning Jesus ... This is how people talk about the manuscript. Thus news gradually comes to light. But the main thing is the extraordinary profundity of the text and the intimate relationship to it of lamas throughout the East! A good and sensitive Indian speaks in a remarkable way about the manuscript, about the life of Issa [Jesus]: "Why is Issa always sent to Egypt during [his] absence from Palestine? The years of his youth were, of course, devoted to study ... It is

---

* *Altai-Himalaya.* Diary of the trans-Himalayan journey of N. Roerich 1925–28, published by *Mysl*, Moscow 1974. All the quotations that follow are taken from chapters 5 and 9.

incomprehensible why Issa's journey on the caravan route to India and to the region we now call Tibet is so fiercely denied!"'

'An old lama-king arrived [from Ladakh] . . . It transpired in the course of conversation that the family of the king knows the manuscripts about Issa. They even said that many Muslims would wish to possess this document.'

And somewhat later, in the same diary, Roerich's reaction to the rumours – which even reached Moscow – that he had finally found the secret manuscript: 'The Moscow papers say that we have "found" the manuscript about Christ [Issa]. Where does this notion come from? How could we find what has long been known? But we have found more. We have been able to establish that the notion of Issa as a member of the community is accepted and lives throughout the East. The text of the manuscript lives on the borders of Bhutan, in Tibet, on the hills of Sikkim, on the heights of Ladakh [that is, in all regions where the Himalayan mahatmas are most in evidence], and in the Mongolian khoshuns [tents] and in the Kalmuck ulus [yurts]. It lives there not as the sensationalism of Sunday newspapers but as a firm and calm awareness. What for the West is sensationalism is for the East ancient knowledge. As one travels through Asia one may become convinced of how these people think.'

Supplement VII. Rudolf Steiner's Notes about the Theosophical Society (see p. 11)

The following notes were written by Rudolf Steiner himself in 1907, while he was staying in Barr (Alsace) as a guest of the French writer and occultist Edouard Schuré at his country home.

Making use of a rare opportunity, Schuré asked his guest three questions: about the spiritual development of Rudolf Steiner himself, about Christian Rosenkreutz and about the Theosophical Society; and he received his answers in written form. This is the reason for their particular trustworthiness, inasmuch as all possibility of inaccurate transmission of meaning or incorrect understanding is completely excluded – which is not the case with lectures recorded in shorthand, still less if they have not been revised by the lecturer.

In 1907 this manuscript, which reveals the occult foundations of the arising and development of the Theosophical movement and the Theosophical Society, was intended solely for Schuré's personal use. Subsequently, however – after his withdrawal from the Theosophical Society – Rudolf Steiner returned on several occasions to this theme in his lectures, especially in 1915 (see GA 254). Thus Rudolf Steiner's literary estate considered it possible in 1967 to publish these notes within the framework of the complete edition of his works (in GA 262); and their final part is reproduced here in its entirety.*

---

* Translation by Christian and Ingrid von Arnim from *Correspondence and Documents 1901–1925, Rudolf Steiner and Marie Steiner-von Sivers*, Rudolf Steiner Press and Anthroposophic Press 1988.

(III)

For information only. It cannot be stated directly in this form at present.

The Theosophical Society was first established in 1875 in New York by H.P. Blavatsky and H.S. Olcott, and had a decidedly western nature. The publication *Isis Unveiled*, in which Blavatsky revealed a large number of esoteric truths, has just such a western character. But it has to be stated regarding this publication that it frequently presents the great truths of which it speaks in a distorted or even caricatured manner. It is similar to a visage of harmonious proportions, appearing distorted in a convex mirror. The things which are said in 'Isis' are true, but *how* they are said is a lopsided mirror-image of the truth. This is because the truths themselves are *inspired* by the great *initiates of the West*, who also inspired the Rosicrucian wisdom.* The distortion arises because of the inappropriate way in which H.P. Blavatsky's *soul* has received these truths. The educated world should have seen in *this* fact alone the evidence for a higher source of inspiration of these truths. For no one who rendered them in such a distorted manner could have created these truths himself. Because the western initiators saw how little opportunity they had to allow the stream of spiritual wisdom to flow into mankind by this means, they decided to drop the matter *in this form* for the time being. But the door had been opened: Blavatsky's soul had been prepared in such a manner that spiritual wisdom was able to

* Rudolf Steiner speaks in many of his lectures about the origin of Blavatsky's *first* great work as springing from Rosicrucian inspirations. See, for example, GA 130, 27 September 1911 and GA 133, 23 October 1911.

flow into it. *Eastern* initiators were able to take hold of her. To begin with these eastern initiators had the best of intentions. They saw how Anglo-American influences were steering mankind towards the terrible danger of a completely materialistic impregnation of thinking. They – these eastern initiators – wanted to imprint *their* form of spiritual knowledge, which had been preserved through the ages, on the western world. Under the influence of this stream the Theosophical Society took on its eastern character, and the same influence was the inspiration for Sinnett's *Esoteric Buddhism* and Blavatsky's *Secret Doctrine*. But both of these became distortions of the truth. Sinnett's work distorts the high teaching of the initiators through an extraneous and inadequate philosophical intellectualism and Blavatsky's *Secret Doctrine* does the same because of her chaotic soul.

The result was that the initators, the eastern ones as well, withdrew their influence in increasing measure from the official Theosophical Society and the latter became the arena for all kinds of occult forces which distorted the great cause. There was a short phase, when Annie Besant entered the stream of initiators through her pure and elevated mentality. But this phase came to an end when Annie Besant gave herself up to the influence of certain Indians who developed a grotesque intellectualism derived from certain philosophical teachings, German ones in particular, which they misinterpreted. This was the situation when I was faced with the necessity of joining the Theosophical Society. True initiators stood at its cradle and *that is why* it is *at present* an instrument of current spiritual life, even if subsequent events have resulted in certain imperfections. Its continued fruitful development in western countries is dependent completely on the extent to which it shows itself capable of assimilating the principle of western initiation among its influences. For the eastern initiations must of necessity leave untouched the *Christ* as the central *cosmic* factor of evolution. But without this principle the theosophical movement will have no decisive influence on western cultures, which trace their beginnings back to Christ's life on Earth. If taken on their own, the revelations of oriental initiation would have to stand aside from the living culture in the West in a sectarian manner. They could only hope for success within evolution if the principle of Christianity were to be eradicated from western culture. But this would be the same as eradicating the essential *meaning of the Earth*, which lies in the recognition and realisation of the intentions of the *living Christ*. To reveal those intentions in the form of complete wisdom, beauty and activity is, however, the deepest aim of Rosicrucianism. Regarding the value of eastern wisdom as the subject of study, one can only say that this study is of the highest value, because western cultures have lost their sense of esotericism, while the eastern ones have preserved theirs. But equally it should be understood that the introduction of a correct esotericism in the West can only be of the Rosicrucian-Christian type, because this *latter* gave birth to western life and because by its loss mankind would deny the meaning and destiny of the Earth.

The harmonious relationship between science and religion can flower only in this esotericism, while every amalgamation of western knowledge with eastern esotericism can only produce such unproductive mongrels as Sinnett's *Esoteric Buddhism*. The correct way can be represented schematically as:

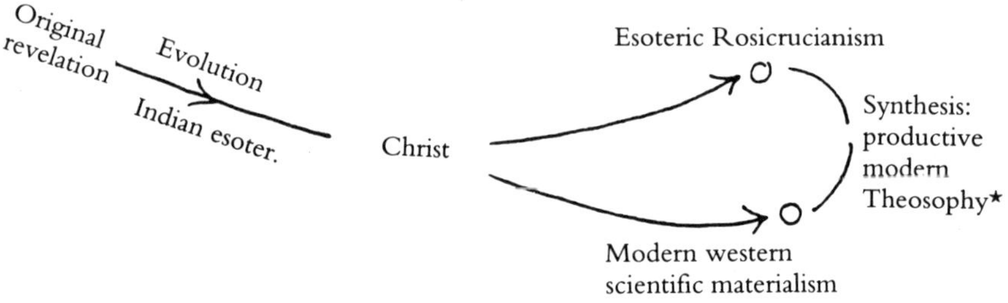

The incorrect way, of which Sinnett's *Esoteric Buddhism* and Blavatsky's *Secret Doctrine* are examples, would be represented as:

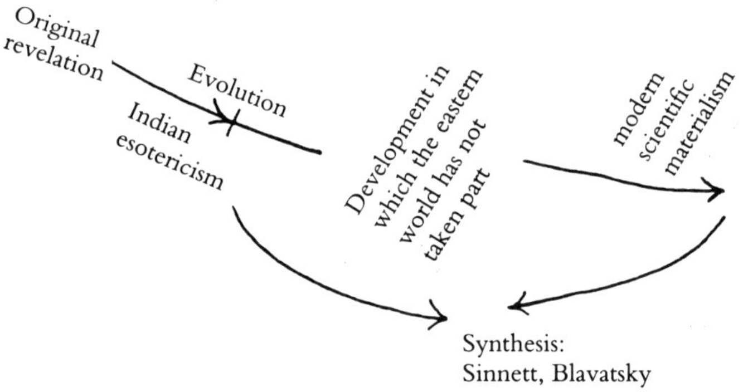

* By 'productive modern Theosophy' is meant Anthroposophy.

Supplement VIII. The Mahatma Letter 'on God' (see p. 43)

The following long excerpt from a letter of the mahatma Kut Humi, which was sent in September 1882 to a friend and colleague of A.P. Sinnett, the Christian A.O. Hume,* bears the title 'Notes by K.H. on a "Preliminary Chapter" headed "God" by Hume, intended to preface an exposition on Occult Philosophy'.

This letter, which is also known in theosophical and Roerich circles as the 'letter about God', might more appropriately be called the 'letter against God'. It is quoted here because of its obvious affinity – as regards both content and style – to Helena Roerich's book *Community* and to the 'Letter of the Mahatmas' to the Bolshevik Government. Thus we have in it a concrete testimony of a consistent and uninterupted flow of development from 1882 to 1927. For in this letter are contained all the foundations of the new understanding of 'religion as the teaching of the all-embracing nature of matter' spoken of in the 'Letter of the Mahatmas' (see p. 37f.) and further developed in *Community*.

On becoming generally familiar with the content of this collection of selected letters from the mahatmas, which were translated into Russian and published by Helena Roerich under the title *Chasha vostoka* ('The Chalice of the East') in 1925 (reprinted in 1926), one is struck that the translator has chosen those letters which are as regards their content espe-

* Published in the volume *The Mahatma Letters to A.P. Sinnett*, third edition, Adyar, Madras, India 1979.

cially close to the book *Community* (whose appearance was in the following year), inasmuch as they often speak of the eternity of matter, of reason as a manifestation of the activity of the brain, of the significance of materialism, of religion, of the source of evil and illusion as begotten of human ignorance – and so on. Many of these utterances are in their style and content strangely reminiscent of certain statements of Marx and Lenin, which in itself lends support to what the mahatmas communicate in *Community*, namely, that their emissaries visited the former in London and the latter in Switzerland (see p. 26).

This choice of letters is, of course, not fortuitous, for according to Helena Roerich she received indications regarding both the translation of the letters into Russian and the content of the book *Community* from one and the same mahatma (though with an interruption of almost a year), whom the Roerichs met in 1925 and then again in 1926, on their way from India to Bolshevik Russia.

After the long quotation from the letter to Hume there follow some short extracts from other letters chosen by Helena Roerich. The number of similar utterances could be considerably augmented without any difficulty.

★

By way of a conclusion to this brief introduction, it is necessary to append a few statements which may serve as a counterbalance to the content of the letter which follows.

In St John's Gospel Christ says: 'God is spirit, and those who worship Him must worship in spirit and in truth' (4:24). And as man was originally created 'in the image and likeness of God' (Genesis 1:27), we should in this same sense understand the following words of the modern Christian initiate, Rudolf Steiner: 'Man is a spirit; and *his* world is the world of spiritual beings' (GA 26, article of 12 October 1924). But the world of spiritual beings is, from the standpoint of Christian esotericism, none other than the world of the nine higher Hierarchies, from the Angels to the Seraphim (see GA 13), with whom – when the ultimate goal of earthly evolution has been attained – human beings will be united as pure spirits to pure spirits, as a new, *tenth* hierarchy, which will represent in our cosmos the principles of *freedom and love* (see GA 110, 18 April 1909 (II)). Thus freedom and love, which in their highest and most spiritual form were revealed to humanity in the Mystery of Golgotha, have since that time come to represent the holiest and most exalted ideals which humanity has on Earth. However, their fulfilment – that is, the fulfilment of '*the intentions of the living Christ*' – is strongly opposed by all forms of the materialism which is being disseminated throughout the cosmos. For 'anyone who speaks out of some world-conception or other about the eternity of matter destroys, on the one hand, freedom and, on the other, a fully developed capacity for love' (GA 202, 19 December 1920). For 'wherever people are lost in contemplation of matter, Ahriman is indeed present' – he who is the greatest opponent of earthly evolution (GA 145, 28 March 1913).

★

Letter No. 10
Notes by K.H. on a 'PRELIMINARY CHAPTER' headed 'GOD' by HUME, intended to preface an EXPOSITION OF OCCULT PHILOSOPHY (abridged).
Received at Simla, Sept. 1882.

Neither our philosophy nor ourselves believe in a God, least of all in one whose pronoun necessitates a capital H.

Our philosophy falls under the definition of Hobbes.* It is pre-eminently the science of effects by their causes and of causes by their effects, and since it is also the science of things deduced from first principle, as Bacon† defines it, before we admit any such principle we must know it, and have no right to admit even its possibility. Your whole explanation is based upon one solitary admission made simply for argument's sake in October last. You were told that our knowledge was limited to this our solar system: ergo as philosophers who desired to remain worthy of the name we could not either deny or affirm the existence of what you termed a supreme, omnipotent, intelligent being of some sort beyond the limits of that solar system. But if such an existence is not absolutely impossible, yet unless the uniformity of nature's laws breaks at those limits we maintain that it is highly improbable. Nevertheless we deny most emphatically the position of agnosticism in this direction, and as regards the solar system. Our doctrine knows no compromises. It either affirms or denies, for it never teaches but that which it knows to be the truth. Therefore, we deny God both as philosophers and as Buddhists. We know there are planetary and other spiritual lives, and we know there is in our system no such thing as God, either personal or impersonal. Parabrahm is not a God, but absolute immutable law, and Iswar‡ is the effect of Avidya and Maya, ignorance based upon the great

* Thomas Hobbes (1588–1679) – English philosopher and materialist, pupil of Francis Bacon. (This and all other footnotes in this Supplement by the Translator.)

† Francis Bacon (1561–1626) – English philosopher, ancestor of English materialism.

‡ Iswar – a concept of Vedantic philosophy, close in meaning to the concept of the 'creative Logos'.

delusion. The word 'God' was invented to designate the unknown cause of those effects which man has either admired or dreaded without understanding them, and since we claim and that we are able to prove what we claim – *i.e.*, the knowledge of that cause and causes – we are in a position to maintain there is no God or Gods behind them.

The idea of God is not an innate but an acquired notion, and we have but one thing in common with theologies – we reveal the infinite. But while we assign to all the phenomena that proceed from the infinite and limitless space, duration and motion, *material, natural, sensible and known* (to us at least) causes, the theists assign them *spiritual, supernatural* and *unintelligible* and un-known causes. The God of the Theologians is simply an imaginary power, *un loup garou* as d'Holbach* expressed it – a power which has never yet manifested itself. Our chief aim is to deliver humanity of this nightmare, to teach man virtue for its own sake, and to walk in life relying on himself instead of leaning on a theological crutch, that for countless ages was the direct cause of nearly all human misery. Pantheistic we may be called – agnostic NEVER. If people are willing to accept and to regard as God our ONE LIFE immutable and unconscious in its eternity they may do so and thus keep to one more gigantic misnomer. But then they will have to say with Spinoza† that there is not and that we cannot conceive any other substance than God; or as that famous and unfortunate philosopher says in his fourteenth proposition,

---

* P.A. d'Holbach (1723–89) – French philosopher. One of the principal founders of French materialism. Criticised religion from a position of extreme atheism.

† B. Spinoza (1632–77) – Dutch philosopher and pantheist. Did not acknowledge Christianity.

'praeter Deum neque dari neque concipi potest substantia' – and thus become Pantheists*... Who but a Theologian nursed on mystery and the most absurd supernaturalism can imagine a self-existent being of necessity infinite and omnipresent *outside* the manifested *boundless* universe. The word infinite is but a negative which excludes the idea of bounds. It is evident that a being independent and omnipresent cannot be limited by anything which is outside of himself; that there can be nothing exterior to himself – not even vacuum, then where is there room for matter? for that manifested universe even though the latter [be] limited? If we ask the theist is your God vacuum, space or matter, they will reply no. And yet they hold that their God penetrates matter though he is not himself matter. When we speak of our One Life we also say that it penetrates, nay is the essence of every atom of matter; and that therefore it not only has correspondence with matter but has all its properties likewise, etc, – hence *is* material, is *matter itself.* How can intelligence proceed or emanate from non-intelligence – you kept asking last year. How could a highly intelligent humanity, man the crown of reason, be evolved out of blind unintelligent law or force! But once we reason on that line, I may ask in my turn, how could congenital idiots, non-reasoning animals, and the rest of 'creation' have been created by or evoluted from, absolute wisdom, if the latter is a thinking intelligent being, the author and ruler of the Universe? How? says Dr Clarke in his examination of the proof of the existence of the Divinity. 'God who hath made the eye, shall he not see? God who hath made the ear, shall he not hear?' But according to this mode of reasoning they would have to admit that in creating an idiot God is an

* Here and subsequently, the ellipses are in the original text.

idiot; that he who made so many irrational beings, so many physical and moral monsters, must be an irrational being. . .

. . .We are not Adwaitees, but our teaching respecting the one life is identical with that of the Adwaitee with regard to Parabrahm. And no true philosophically trained Adwaitee will ever call himself an agnostic, for he knows that he is Parabrahm and identical in every respect with the universal life and soul – the macrocosm is the microcosm and he knows that there is no God apart from himself, no creator as no being. Having found Gnosis we cannot turn our backs on it and become agnostics.

. . .Were we to admit that even the highest Dhyan Chohans are liable to err under a delusion, then there would be no reality for us indeed and the occult sciences would be as great a chimera as that God. If there is an absurdity in denying that which we do not know it is still more extravagant to assign to it unknown laws.

According to logic 'nothing' is that of which everything can truly be denied and nothing can truly be affirmed. The idea therefore either of a finite or infinite nothing is a contradiction in terms. And yet according to theologians 'God, the self existent being is a most simple, unchangeable, incorruptible being; without parts, figure, motion, divisibility, or any other such properties as we find in matter. For all such things so plainly and necessarily imply finiteness in their very notion and are utterly inconsistent with complete infinity.' Therefore the God here offered to the adoration of the 19th century lacks every quality upon which man's mind is capable of fixing any judgement. What is this in fact but a being of whom they can affirm *nothing* that is not instantly contradicted. Their own Bible, their Revelation, destroys all the moral perfections they heap upon him, unless indeed they call those qualities

> perfections that every other man's reason and common sense call imperfections, odious vices and brutal wickedness. Nay more, he who reads our Buddhist scriptures written for the superstitious masses will fail to find in them a *demon* so vindictive, unjust, so cruel and so stupid as the celestial tyrant upon which the Christians prodigally lavish their servile worship and on whom their theologians heap those perfections that are contradicted on every page of their Bible. Truly and veritably your theology has created her God but to destroy him piecemeal. Your church is the fabulous Saturn, who begets children but to devour them.

There then follow some answers to certain questions posed to the mahatma by Hume in his letters:

> A few reflections and arguments ought to support every new idea – for instance we are sure to be taken to task for the following apparent contradictions. (1) We deny the existence of a thinking conscious God, on the grounds that such a God must either be conditioned, limited and subject to change, therefore not infinite, or (2) he is represented to us as an eternal unchangeable and independent being, with not a particle of matter in him, then we answer that it is no being but an immutable blind principle, a law. And yet, they will say, we believe in Dhyans, or Planetaries ('spirits' also), and endow them with a universal mind, *and this must be explained.*
>
> Our reasons may be briefly summed up thus:
>
> (1) We deny the absurd proposition that there can be, even in a boundless and eternal universe – two infinite eternal and omnipresent existences.
>
> (2) Matter we know to be eternal, *i.e.*, having had no

beginning (a) because matter is Nature herself (b) because that which cannot annihilate itself and is indestructible exists necessarily – and therefore it could not begin to be, not can it cease to be (c) because the accumulated experience of countless ages, and that of exact science show to us matter (or nature) acting by her own peculiar energy, of which not an atom is ever in an absolute state of rest, and therefore it must have always existed, *i.e.*, its materials ever changing form, combinations and properties, but its principles or elements being absolutely indestructible.
(3) As to God – since no one has ever or at any time seen him or it – *unless he or it is the very essence and nature of this boundless eternal matter, its energy and motion*, we cannot regard him as either eternal or infinite or yet self existing. We refuse to admit a being or an existence of which we know absolutely nothing; because (a) there is no room for him in the presence of that matter whose undeniable properties and qualities we know thoroughly well (b) because if he or it is but a part of that matter it is ridiculous to maintain that he is the mover and ruler of that of which he is but a dependent part and (c) because if they tell us that God is a self existent pure spirit independent of matter – an extra-cosmic deity, we answer that admitting even the possibility of such an impossibility, *i.e.*, his existence, we yet hold that a purely immaterial spirit cannot be an intelligent conscious ruler nor can he have any of the attributes bestowed upon him by theology, and thus such a God becomes again but a blind force. Intelligence, as found in our Dhyans Chohans, is a faculty that can appertain but to organized or animated being – however imponderable or rather *invisible* the materials of their organizations. Intelligence requires the necessity of thinking; to think one must have ideas; ideas suppose senses which are physical material,

and how can anything material belong to pure spirit? If it be objected that thought cannot be a property of matter, we will ask the reason why? We must have an unanswerable proof of this assumption, before we can accept it. Of the theologian we would enquire what was there to prevent his God, since he is the alleged creator of all – to endow matter with the faculty of thought; and when answered that evidently it has not pleased Him to do so, that it is a mystery as well as an impossibility, we would insist upon being told why it is more impossible that matter should produce spirit and thought, than spirit or the thought of God should produce and create matter.

We do not bow our heads in the dust before the mystery of mind – for we *have solved it ages ago*. Rejecting with contempt the theistic theory we reject as much the automation theory, teaching that states of consciousness are produced by the marshalling of the molecules of the brain; and we feel as little respect for that other hypothesis – the production of molecular motion by consciousness. Then what do we believe in? Well, we believe in the much laughed at *phlogiston* (see article 'What is force and what is matter?' *Theosophist*, September), and in what some natural philosophers would call *nisus*, the incessant though perfectly imperceptible (to the ordinary senses) motion or efforts one body is making on another – the pulsations of inert matter – its life. The bodies of the Planetary spirits are formed of that which Priestley* and others called Phlogiston and for which we have another name – the essence in its highest seventh state forming that matter of which the organisms of the highest and purest Dhyans are composed, and in its lowest or densest form (so impalpable yet that

* Joseph Priestley (1733–1804) – English chemist and philosopher.

> science calls it energy and force) serving as a cover to the Planetaries of the 1st or lowest degree. In other words we believe in matter alone, in *matter* as visible nature and matter in its invisibility as the invisible omnipresent omnipotent Proteus with its unceasing motion which is its life, and which nature draws from herself since she is the great whole outside of which nothing can exist. For as Bilfinger* truly asserts, motion is a manner of existence that flows necessarily out of the essence of matter; that matter moves by its own peculiar energies; that its motion is due to the force which is inherent in itself, that the variety of motion and the phenomena that result proceed from the diversity of the properties of the qualities and of the combinations which are originally found in the primitive matter of which nature is the assemblage and of which your science knows less than one of our Tibetan Yak-drivers of Kant's metaphysics.†
>
> The existence of matter then is a fact; the existence of motion is another fact, their self existence and eternity or indestructibility is a third fact. And the idea of pure spirit as a Being or an Existence – give it whatever name you will – is a chimera, a gigantic absurdity.

The letter ends with the mahatmas' views on evil. They see one third of the problem in man himself, in his selfishness, and the other two thirds in religion.

> ...Therefore it is neither nature nor an imaginary Deity that has to be blamed, but human nature made vile by

---

* Bilfinger (1693–1750) – German academic, professor of philosophy and teacher of mathematics.

† Immanuel Kant (1724–1804) – German philosopher.

selfishness. Think well over these few words; work out every cause of evil you can think of and trace it to its origin and you will have solved *one-third* of the problem of evil. And now, after making due allowance for evils that are natural and cannot be avoided, – and so few are they that I challenge the whole host of Western metaphysicians to call them evils or to trace them directly to an independent cause – I will point out the greatest, the chief cause of nearly two thirds of the evils that pursue humanity ever since that cause became a power. It is religion under whatever form and in whatsoever nation. It is the sacerdotal caste, the priesthood and the churches, it is in those illusions that man looks upon as sacred, that he has to search out the source of that multitude of evils which is the greatest curse of humanity and that almost overwhelms mankind. Ignorance created Gods and cunning took advantage of the opportunity. Look at India and look at Christendom and Islam, at Judaism and Fetichism. It is priestly imposture that rendered these Gods so terrible to man; it is religion that makes of him the selfish bigot, the fanatic that hates all mankind out of his own sect without rendering him any better or more moral for it. It is belief in God and Gods that makes two-thirds of humanity the slaves of a handful of those who deceive them under the false pretence of saving them. Is not man ever ready to commit any kind of evil if told that his God or Gods demand the crime – voluntary victim of an illusionary God, the abject slave of his crafty ministers? The Irish, Italian and Slavonian peasant will starve himself and see his family starving and naked to feed and clothe his padre and pope. For two thousand years India groaned under the weight of caste, Brahmins alone feeding on the fat of the land, and to-day the followers of Christ and those of Mahomet are cutting each other's throats in the names of

> and for the greater glory of their respective myths. Remember the sum of human misery will never be diminished unto that day when the better portion of humanity destroys in the name of Truth, morality, and universal charity, the altars of their false gods.
>
> If it is objected to that we too have temples, we too have priests and that our lamas also live on charity . . . let them know that the objects above named have in common with their Western equivalents but the name. Thus in our temples there is neither a god nor gods worshipped, only the thrice sacred memory of the greatest as the holiest man that ever lived [Buddha].

At the end of the letter there follows a long extract from the Buddhist canon, culminating in the words of 'the Fully Enlightened One' [the Buddha]: 'From ignorance spring all evils'.

In conclusion, here are some extracts from other letters:

(Letter IX):

> For I trust you have given up the queer idea – a natural result of early Christian training – that there can possibly be *human* intelligences inhabiting *purely spiritual* regions.
>
> However ethereal and purified of gross matter they may be, the pure Spirits are still subject to the physical and universal laws of matter.

(Letter XIII from M.M.):

> Your 'Lord God', says Bible, chapter I, verses 25 and 26 – after having made *all* said: 'Let us make man in our image,' etc., and creates man – an *androgyne ape*! (extinct on our planet) the highest in intelligence in the animal kingdom and whose descendants you find in the anthropoids of to-day.

(Letter XXII):

... we say this perpetual motion is the only eternal and uncreated Deity we are able to recognise. But of that which lies within the worlds and systems, not in the trans-infinitude – (a queer expression to use) – but in the cis-infinitude rather, in the state of the purest and inconceivable immateriality, no one ever knew or will ever tell, hence it is something non-existent for the universe. You are at liberty to place in this eternal vacuum the intellectual or voluntary powers of your deity – if you can conceive of such a thing.

A pure yet volitional Spirit is an absurdity for volitional mind. The result of organism cannot exist independently of an organized brain, and an organized brain made out of nihil is a still greater fallacy. If you ask me 'Whence then the immutable laws? – laws cannot make themselves' – then in my turn I will ask you – and whence their supposed Creator? – a creator cannot create or make himself. If the brain did not make itself, for this would be affirming that brain acted before it existed, how could intelligence, the result of an organized brain, act before its creator was made?

The conception of matter and spirit as entirely distinct, and both eternal, could certainly never have entered my head, however little I may know of them, for it is one of the elementary and fundamental doctrines of Occultism that the two are one, and are distinct but in their respective manifestations, and only in the limited perceptions of the world of senses.

... matter *per se* is indestructible, and, as I maintain, coeval with spirit – that spirit which we know and can conceive of.

(Letter 23 B):

> Spirit, life and matter, are not natural principles existing independently of each other, but the effects of combinations produced by eternal motion in space.

Appendix

Nicholas and Helena Roerich as Representatives of Occult Bolshevism

As is fully clear from the content of the present book, one of the principal qualities shared by the Roerichs was a deeply positive attitude to Bolshevism in Russia and above all to its leader and chief ideologue – Lenin. From a certain moment and until the very end of their lives this positive attitude remained unchanged, and even the passage of decades was not able to affect it in the slightest.

However, Helena and Nicholas Roerich did not immediately come to such a complete and unqualified acceptance of Leninist Bolshevism. To begin with, after the October Revolution of 1917, guided by the natural feelings of educated and culture-loving people, they had a negative attitude to the Bolsheviks' seizure of power, reckoning them to be barbarians and destroyers of all culture. Only after their meeting in London in 1920 with that individuality whom they were subsequently to venerate as their spiritual teacher did their opinion of the Bolsheviks and of everything that was taking place in Russia change completely.

As was pointed out in the footnote on p. 14, it is not the task of the present study to investigate the question as to *who* that individuality whom the Roerichs, after their meeting with him, always called 'Mahatma M'. (Morya) really was. Whether he was the occultist of the Eastern path who bore this name, of whom much was said in theosophical circles in the time of Blavatsky, or a completely different individuality who had merely adopted a name that was not his own – this question lies beyond the compass of this book. Of greater importance here is the fact that the Roerichs were absolutely convinced that the individuality who had made contact with them was Mahatma Morya, and everything that they did and wrote after their meeting with him was done and written according to his instructions and with his agreement.

In the weekly journal *Znamya mira* ('Banner of Peace') recently founded in Moscow by the adherents of Agni Yoga, in one of the numbers for April 1993, an article appeared – according to the editorship only the first of a whole series – which was devoted to a study of Lenin's mission from the standpoint of Agni Yoga. The article is accompanied by a portrait of the leader, and its title is a quotation from Helena Roerich's book *Community*: 'Take the appearance of Lenin as a sign of the sensitivity of the cosmos' – an unambiguous indication of the 'cosmic' dimensions of his mission.

In the article there appear the following words: 'The Mission of Vladimir Ilich Lenin (Ulyanov) is so complex that even the Roerichs were only able to understand it from the Highest Plane. It is known that even in 1919 N.K. Roerich supposed the Bolsheviks to be "destroyers of culture". It is also known that after 24 March 1920 the Roerichs became ardent "reds" [that is, Bolshevik in their sympathies]. On this day there took place their meeting with Mahatma M. Evidently, their initiation into the Plan of the Rulers [the mahatmas] had begun.'[1]

And then the author of the article turns to a question put by him to an old pupil of N.K. Roerich: 'How can the New Epoch and the coercive means of inaugurating the new order in 1917 be reconciled with one another?' The pupil's answer was brief and clear: 'Not to accept Lenin's Mission is not to accept the Plan of the Rulers [the mahatmas]'.

However people today may relate to these words, spoken at the end of 1989, they could when applied to the Roerichs fully serve as a leitmotif of their entire lives *after* their first meeting with the mahatma.

Indeed, already in 1924 Helena Roerich – while she was abroad – brought out the first volume of *Agni Yoga* under the title, *Listy sada Morya* ('Leaves of Morya's Garden'), part I, *Zov* ('The Call').[2] On the second page of the book a date is given: 'London. March 24th, 1920' – that is, the day of the meeting with the mahatma; and on the first page the words with which the book itself begins: 'To the new Russia – My first proclamation'.*[3] The word 'My' is printed with a capital and refers to the mahatma who – according to Helena Roerich's conviction – dictated to her not only this first but also all the subsequent thirteen volumes of *Agni Yoga* by mediumistic means.

In 1921, again abroad, Nicholas Roerich published a collection of his poems. In its title the name of Mahatma M... is again contained: *Tsvyety Morii* ('Flowers of Morya').[4] The author prefaces the poems with an epigraph, which begins with the words: 'Above all other Russias is the one Russia which will endure'. In the context of the above-quoted words dictated to Helena Roerich by Mahatma M., what is meant here too is the 'new', that is, Bolshevik Russia.

The Roerichs henceforth had to serve this new Russia, and in 1926 their spiritual teacher sent them to its rulers. On the way there, while they were crossing the Himalayas, he dictated to Helena Roerich the third volume of *Agni Yoga*,

---

* Subsequent foreign editions of Helena Roerich's works, obviously not wishing to compromise themselves by openly manifesting sympathy for the Bolsheviks, generally omitted or metamorphosed this first phrase.

Obshchina (*Community*), together with the letter to the Bolshevik Government, which the Roerichs were to pass on to its representatives in Moscow. Then the same mahatma ordered the Roerichs to return to India via Mongolia, where they were also entrusted with carrying out a certain task (see p. 45).

In the Mongolian capital of Ulan-Bator, Helena Roerich personally published the text of *Community* in Russian (anonymously, without any indication of the author's name)*[5] in a small edition of 200–300 copies. It is, therefore, this edition – now a bibliographical rarity – which most precisely and directly transmits everything said by the mahatma to Helena Roerich in the Himalayas. The Mongolian edition has the subtitle: 'Leaves of Conversations of the High Member of the Community of the East' and is a direct continuation of the first two books of *Agni Yoga*: *The Call* and *Illumination*, which have the common title of *Leaves of Morya's Garden*.

The authorship of the same mahatma standing *behind all three books* is confirmed by the beginning of the next, fourth volume, which appeared in 1929 under the title *Znaki Agni-yogi* ('Signs of Agni Yoga'). There we read the words: 'The revered Mahatma, who gave the books *The Call*, *Illumination* and *Community* transmitted the many counsels and signs of Agni Yoga. These practical indications have been collected by us for the use of those who seek knowledge.'[6] And in *Community* the relationship between these first three books is spoken of as follows: 'The book *The Call* knew no impediments. The book *Illumination* is like a stone. The book

---

* This anonymity, apart from possible considerations of personal safety, had above all an occult significance. For Helena Roerich considered that the author of this and all the subsequent books of *Agni Yoga* was not herself but the mahatma who dictated their content to her.

Community is like someone sailing against a storm, where every sail and every rope sustain life.'[7]

It was in *Community*, which was first dictated by the Eastern mahatma and then, in accordance with his indication, published in the Mongolian capital, that all the highly positive statements about Lenin, Bolshevism and its materialistic world-view are contained, some of which have already been cited in the present work (see p. 39f.). That the mahatmas also caused some Himalayan soil to be brought through the Roerichs to Lenin's grave gives the stamp of ratification and confirms the autheniticity of all these statements.

During her stay in Mongolia Helena Roerich anonymously, and also in Russian, published one further book, *Osnovy Buddizma* (*The Foundations of Buddhism*).[8] In it can be found a whole series of thoughts which almost literally coincide with many places in *Community*. For example, she writes of Gautama Buddha that he was a 'fighter for community and matter', or that 'in the teachings of Buddha we find . . . materialistic philosophy', 'the living creativity of great matter'. There one can also read that Buddha 'attained to a premonition of the Maitreya – the symbol of the age of knowledge about the greatness of matter. . .' Finally, in the same book, Helena Roerich cites a long quotation from a certain professor from Petrograd (his name is not given), who gave expression in his lecture to a 'universe without God' and called this one of the basic features 'both of Buddhist and of our modern, most recent [meaning Bolshevik] world-conception', a view with which Helena Roerich wholly agrees, criticising in the section that she quotes only the pupil's denial of freedom of the will but not his denial of God.

Only when the task of the mahatmas had been accomplished and both books were published did the Roerichs leave Ulan-Bator and follow the caravan road to the south, back to

India. This took place on 13 April 1927. The same year is also of significance as the year of the first edition in a jacket of *Community*. Subsequently, however, on its republication in Europe in 1936 the year 1926 was inscribed on it,[9] which refers not to the year of the book's first publication but to the year of its dictation by the mahatma.

If we turn from a reading of *Community* and *The Foundations of Buddhism* to the 'Letter of the Mahatmas' to the Bolshevik Government (see p. 37f.), we may be particularly struck by their similar style, even to the extent that in some places there are individual expressions and turns of phrase which correspond with the text of *Community*. So there is little doubt that both documents, the book and the letter, were composed by one and the same personality and at approximately the same time. This was indeed the case. As has been said, both the letter and *Community* were dictated by the mahatma to Helena Roerich at the end of 1925 and the beginning of 1926 during the expedition from India to Russia.

Thus in *Community* reference is made to 'the particular criminality of the church, which is a repository of dark traditions', to the need to 'strengthen [in schools] the lines of materially authentic knowledge'; also to 'pseudo-communists', who 'must be avoided like an infection of syphilis', to 'the dissemination of vanity, ignorance and fear', to the overcoming of the dark legacy of the past; then to the battle against hypocrisy and falsehood (of course with those who sully the radiant form of Leninist Communism); and again and again mention is made of the significance of matter and materialism as the principal forces of the epoch that is to come, by which is meant its higher religion, and so on. Both as regards its content and its style (highly reminiscent of the headlines of Bolshevik newspapers and especially of the writings of Lenin himself), *Community* is none other than an expanded commentary to the 'Letter of the Mahatmas' to the Bolshevik Government and – in all essentials – forms with it a single whole.

In his acknowledgement of Lenin as a cosmic phenomenon Nicholas Roerich was the equal of Helena. In 1926 he wrote: 'He [Lenin] incorporated and circumspectly fitted every material into the world order. This opened up to him the path into all parts of the world. And people have formed a legend not only as a record of his deeds but also as a mark of his aspirations. Behind us lie twenty-four countries [he here refers to all the countries through which the Roerichs have travelled, especially those in Asia], and we have seen for ourselves how the nations have understood the magnetic power of communism. Friends, the worst counsellor is negativity. Behind every negation ignorance is concealed. And in ignorance is the hydra of counter-revolution.'[10]

These words were most likely written by Roerich during his stay in Bolshevik Russia. Shortly before this, while he was in Urumchi – within the territory of China – awaiting permission to depart, he wrote in his diary some words of E. Chin-Ben, who on the occasion of Lenin's death compared him with no less than 'Shakya-Muni [Buddha] and Christ'. Roerich was in complete agreement with this, and for this called its author a 'light-filled, brave and honourable Chinaman'.[11]

This frank acknowledgement of the rightness of such a comparison represents the culmination of the relationship between the Roerichs and Lenin. Despite its blasphemous character and its obvious absurdity, it is fully compatible with the content of *Community*, where Lenin is spoken of as a cosmic phenomenon ('a sign of the sensitivity of the cosmos'), and with the 'Letter of the Mahatmas' to the Bolshevik Government and, finally, with the Himalayan soil brought by them for the grave of 'Mahatma Lenin'.

It is true that Helena Roerich made some significant revisions to *Community* for its republication in Riga (1936) and removed the most pro-communist portions, which is, however, wholly understandable. For to bring it out openly in Europe and America in the mid-1930s with its adulations of Lenin and the Bolsheviks without ruining her reputation and being branded as an 'agent of the Reds' was virtually impossible.

On the other hand, the Roerichs' followers in Russia tried several times after the so-called Krushchev thaw to publish material about the relationship of the Roerichs to Lenin, with the object of proving the complete loyalty of the founders of Agni Yoga to the ruling regime. They hoped thereby to gain for themselves the possibility of a more legal existence and indeed made some progress in this respect.

As for the Roerichs, subsequent years did not fundamentally alter their relationship to Lenin's mission and to Bolshevism. As testimony of this there are not only their fairly numerous letters and diary entries from the 1930s and 1940s, some of which have already been cited in the present book (see p. 48) but above all their deeply rooted family tradition.

Thus many years after the death of Helena and Nicholas Roerich, their youngest son and sole heir, Svyatoslav (died 1993), true to this family tradition, in November 1989 made the Roerichs' followers in Moscow a 'valuable' gift. He personally presented them from his father's library in India with a very rare copy of the first – Mongolian – edition of *Community*, signing it with his own hand (see the reproduction of the book's cover on p. 158). The fact of this gift, made *after* the fall of Bolshevism in Russia, is an eloquent testimony of the faithfulness of *all* the members of the Roerich family until the very end of their lives to the 'Mission of Lenin'. And indeed, how could this be otherwise, if its 'cosmic' significance was once revealed to Helena and Nicholas Roerich by their spiritual leader, the mahatma himself?

This unique copy was in the following year (1990) reproduced in Moscow by the Roerichs' followers. V. Sidorov – the President of the Commission for the Literary Legacy of N.K. Roerich – wrote a foreword for it, the title of which consisted of words from *Community*: 'Don't miss the boat!' Sidorov's foreword begins with the words: 'In June 1926 in the Kremlin there took place a ceremony of presentation to the People's Commissar for Foreign Affairs, Chicherin, of a letter from the mahatmas, spiritual leaders and teachers of the East. The Russian artist Nicholas Konstantinovich Roerich, who at that time had gained world renown, presented the letter. In the document, unconditional support was expressed to the new order which had been engendered out of the fire of the revolution: "we have recognised the timeliness of your movement and send you all our help in affirmation of the Oneness of Asia".'

These words, which were written by a well-known pupil of Roerich in the post-Bolshevist era, are perhaps the best reflection of the present mood of the pupils and followers of N. and H. Roerich in Russia who wish – despite all the terrible lessons of history – to remain faithful to the end to the legacy of the founders of Agni Yoga. And whereas in the West their followers do, as a rule, keep an embarrassed silence about the open sympathy of the Roerichs for Bolshevism, thus not only manifesting an inner inconsistency but quite fundamentally deluding the Western public, in Russia the Roerichs' pupils abide by this legacy even now and continue to view it as the substance of what the mahatmas indicated through the Roerichs.

For if we turn to the context out of which Sidorov took the

title for his introductory article, it speaks for itself and further commentaries are unnecessary. Sidorov concludes his foreword with it. 'As pupils of Lenin, watch with an eagle eye, and with the leap of a lion claim the power that is yours. Do not miss the boat!'[12]

★

To conclude this appendix, which has led the reader back to the occult sources of Bolshevism and to the relationship to it and to its founder of the Eastern occultists,[13] it is necessary to speak also about the relationship to it of Western, that is, Christian-Rosicrucian occultism as represented in the 20th century by Rudolf Steiner.

Thus only a year after the Bolsheviks came to power in Russia, Rudolf Steiner indicated 'that in them [Lenin and Trotsky] the greatest, most intense enemies of the spiritual evolution of mankind could be seen',[14] in whom 'there lives ... hatred for the supersensible, even if this comes to expression ... in other words.'[15]

Subsequently, as he gazed ever deeper into the Russian tragedy, Rudolf Steiner in 1919 came to pronounce an even sterner sentence. He called Lenin 'the hangman' and 'grave-digger of all spiritual life', in whom was manifested the aspiration towards 'wild destruction of everything of a spiritual nature'.[16] And then in the same year: 'I know that what lies at the foundation of his [Lenin's] view of the world is not the creating of a new culture but the murder of a culture'.[17] A year later he explains this destructive power of Bolshevism in the following way: 'Bolshevism is so destructive for mankind because it is a creed purely of the brain, the *material* brain',[18] that is, of matter alone. This thought has much in common with these words from *Community*: 'In our acts and our thoughts we cannot separate ourselves from matter', after which one is told about the need for 'a training in the materiality of thinking'.

In the ceremony of handing over the Himalayan soil for Lenin's grave together with the 'Letter of the Mahatmas', the participants on the part of the Soviet Government included – in addition to the Minister for Foreign Affairs, Chicherin – the Minister of Culture, Lunacharsky, with whom the Roerichs had many hours of conversations. If we take the mahatmas' ideas on education (cited on p. 41f.) into consideration, the following words of Rudolf Steiner acquire a special significance: '... Lunacharsky's educational reform is something quite terrible. It is the death of all culture! And although so much that is bad has already emerged from the rest of Bolshevism, the worst will be the Bolshevist methods of education.'[19]

Rudolf Steiner gives the following characterisation of what awaits our Earth in the event of the universal spread of Leninism: 'Mankind would then, beginning with Russia, be mechanised in spirit, vegetabilised in soul and animalised in body',[20] as a result of which all 'human society over the entire Earth would necessarily be transformed into a herd of animals *with no more than a refined thinking capacity*.'[21] For 'in Leninism the *cleverness of the human animal*, the cleverness of the human animality, comes to the surface of human evolution'.

Finally, Rudolf Steiner touches upon the occult nature of Bolshevism. He says: 'Lenin, Trotsky and others like them *are the tools of ahrimanic powers*. This is an ahrimanic initiation, which quite simply *belongs to a different cosmic sphere from ours*. But it is an initiation which bears in its depths the power to efface human civilisation from the Earth, to wipe out everything that has been formed by way of human civilisation.' (Cf. Rudolf Steiner's words about the reasons for the so positive relationship of Eastern initiates to Bolshevism quoted on p. 50).

What do these words of the modern Christian initiate about 'Bolshevist initiation' belonging to 'another cosmic sphere' from the human sphere signify? To what *subhuman* sphere does it belong? The answer to this question has already been given in the pages of this book. Bolshevik initiation has its origin in and is inspired out of *the eighth sphere* and would lead the whole of earthly evolution to it.[22]

Thus already in 1919 Rudolf Steiner said that 'if things were to go further in the way that they have now begun in Russia, this would signify that the Earth would lose its task, would be deprived of its task, would be wrested from the universe and be ahrimanised'.[23]

Rudolf Steiner similarly calls 'Leninism ... the ahrimanic form of anti-Christianity'.[24]

Bearing in mind what has been said, it is not difficult to understand that Bolshevism as a social and occult phenomenon is – first and foremost – deeply alien to all the true tasks of Russia, to the whole of its future mission in the evolution of humanity. Rudolf Steiner referred also to this in 1918, when he said that 'never have such great contrasts collided with one another than the soul of the European East and the anti-humanity of Trotskyism and Leninism'.[25] And two years later he formulated this thought as follows: 'There are many people who think that what is to arise in the East has something to do with Leninism and Trotskyism. They have nothing whatever to do with what is to arise in the East [of Europe] but only with what will perish there and what will be further doomed to perish because of Leninism and Trotskyism. These are purely destructive forces, and what is to arise in the East [of Europe] must develop there in spite of these destructive forces.'[26]

'There are many people...' Amongst these 'many people' were the whole Roerich family, who were misled by the

Tibetan mahatma and who until the very end of their lives preserved an unshakeable belief in the deep-down affinity between Bolshevism and the true tasks of Russia.

All their lives they wanted not to 'miss the boat', but that is exactly what they did.

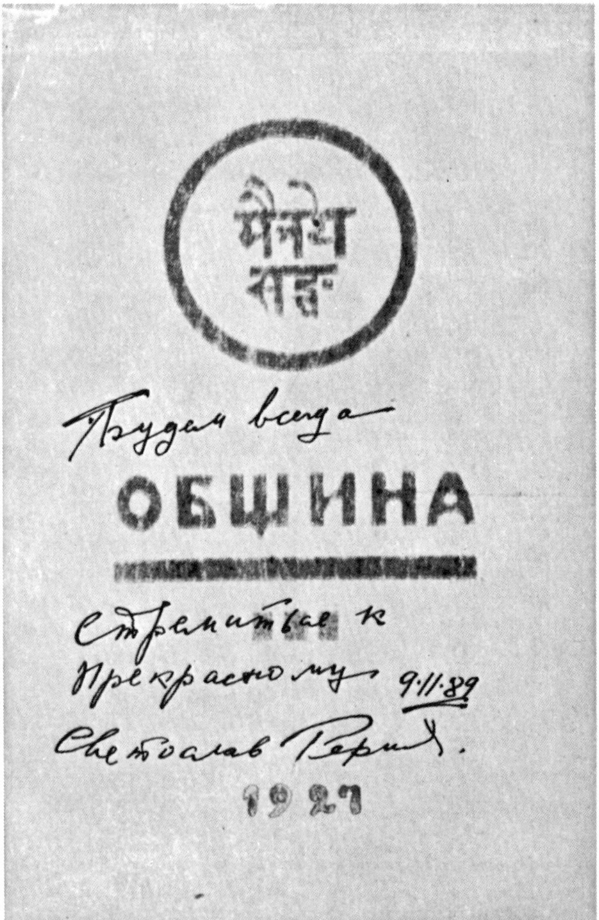

Facsimile of the cover of the first edition of *Community*, signed by Svyatoslav Roerich

Notes

Translator's note: Nicholas and Helena Roerich wrote almost exclusively in Russian, and where their writings are quoted by the author of the present book they have been newly translated from the original Russian text, even where the initial publication was in English (although for ease of reference the titles of the published English translations are given). Readers wishing to consult such published English translations of these writings as are available are warned that in some cases the English editions contain omissions or have been abridged in some way (most strikingly in the case of the book *Community*).

List of Abbreviations

EP	E. Polyakova, *Nikolai Roerich*, Iskusstvo, Moscow 1985.
PB	P. Belikov, V. Knyazeva, *Roerich*, Molodaya gvardiya, Moscow 1973, in the series 'Lives of prominent people'.
NR	*Zazhigaitye serdtse* ('Enkindle the Heart'). Collection of articles and letters from the early years of Nicholas Roerich, Molodaya gvardiya, Moscow 1978.
HR I	Helena Roerich, *Letters 1929–38, vol. I*, Riga 1940.
HR II	Helena Roerich, *Letters 1929–38, vol. II*, Riga 1940.
LMG	Helena Roerich, *Leaves of Morya's Garden*, from the Complete Edition of all 14 books of *Agni Yoga* in three volumes, vol. I, Samara 1992.
AY	Helena Roerich, *Agni Yoga*. Complete Edition of all 14 books in three volumes, Samara 1992.
COM	Helena Roerich, *Community, Agni Yoga vol. III*. Reprint of the first Ulan-Bator edition of 1927 in the journal *Triesvozt, Cultura*, Moscow, Nos. 10–12, 1989 and Nos. 1–10, 1990.
FM	Nicholas Roerich, *Flowers of Morya*. Collection of poems. Khudozhestvyennaya literatura, Moscow 1984.

UG *Uguns* – journal published in the Latvian and Russian languages by the Latvian Roerich Society. Anniversary number, published in January 1990 on the occasion of the 115th anniversary of N. Roerich's birth.

MON The monograph, *Nicholas Roerich. The Life and Work of a Russian Master* by Jacqueline Decter, in collaboration with the Nicholas Roerich Museum, Thames and Hudson, London 1989.

All works by Rudolf Steiner are referred to by the *Gesamtausgabe* (GA) volume number from the catalogue of the collected edition of Rudolf Steiner's works in the original German (published by *Rudolf Steiner Verlag*, Dornach, Switzerland). For information on the published English language translations see the list on page 168.

1. *Pravda*, issue of 15 May 1987. In this issue there is also a photograph of Gorbachev receiving Svyatoslav Roerich at the Kremlin.
2. The quotation is taken from an article by L. Shaposhnikova, *Mudrost vyekov* ('Wisdom of the Ages'), in the journal, *Nauka i religiya* ('Science and Religion'), 2 February1990.
3. From the brochure about *MON* published by *Sphinx* publishing house, Switzerland (Sphinx Medien Verlag, Basel 1989).
4. *MON.*
5. Ibid.
6. See Supplement VII.
7. See the lecture of 6 October 1911 (GA 131).
8. See Supplement VII.
9. Ibid.
10. Lecture of 12 April 1909 (i), GA 110.
11. See Supplement VII.
12. Lecture of 11 October 1915 (GA 254). The next two quotations are from the same source.
13. Ibid., lecture of 18 October 1915.
14. Ibid., lecture of 17 October 1915.
15. Ibid., lecture of 19 October 1915.
16. Ibid., lecture of 17 October 1915.
17. Ibid.
18. Ibid.

19. Ibid.
20. Ibid.
21. Ibid., lecture of 18 October 1915.
22. See Supplement VII.
23. GA 254, lecture of 18 October 1915.
24. Ibid.
25. Lecture of 27 November 1916 (GA 172).
26. *FM.*
27. *AY.*
28. *HR II*, 31 July 1937.
29. Ibid.
30. *LMG* (similarly the quotations that follow).
31. *HR I*, 21 May 1935.
32. *AY.*
33. *UG*, Article by Nicholas Roerich entitled 'Radiant Shamballa'.
34. *AY.*
35. *COM.*
36. *COM* (as with the quotations that follow).
37. Regarding the secret societies of the West and their part in preparing the 'socialist experiment' in Russia which began with the Bolshevist Revolution of 1917, see further in the present author's book, *The Spiritual Origins of Eastern Europe and the Future Mysteries of the Holy Grail*, Temple Lodge Publishing 1993. There will also be found most of Rudolf Steiner's observations on this subject.
38. *PB.*
39. Ibid.
40. See note 37.
41. GA 195, lecture of 1 January 1920.
42. Quoted from *EP.*
43. *PB.*
44. *PB.*
45. N. Roerich, *Altai-Himalaya*, travel diary of 1925–1928, published by Mysl, Moscow 1974.
46. *EP.*
47. Quoted in *EP.*
48. *EP.*

49. *COM* (similarly with the quotations that follow).
50. For an introduction to the pedagogy founded upon the anthroposophical view of man, see *Education towards Freedom* (English edition published by Lanthorn Press, 1976; Russian edition published in Moscow, 1993.)
51. *HR I*, 12 September 1934. See Supplement VIII.
52. Ibid.
53. *HR II*, 4 June 1937.
54. *HR II*, 24 May 1936.
55. *EP*.
56. *PB*.
57. See note 45.
58. *HR II*, 17 December 1935.
59. *NR*.
60. Ibid.
61. Ibid.
62. *COM*.
63. GA 196, lecture of 9 January 1920.
64. *HR I*, 21 May 1935.
65. *HR II*, 3 December 1937 and 5 April 1938.
66. See Rudolf Steiner's *Occult Science – An Outline* (GA 13), the chapter entitled 'Evolution of the World and of Man'.
67. *HR II*, 3 December 1937.
68. *COM*.
69. Similar descriptions can be found in the books of A. Besant and C. Leadbeater.
70. GA 201, lecture of 16 April 1920.
71. GA 258, lecture of 15 June 1923.
72. *HR I*, 1 February 1935.
73. GA 254, lecture of 18 October 1915.
74. Ibid., as with the quotations that follow.
75. *AY*.
76. Helena Roerich's words are quoted in V. Sidorov's foreword to *COM*.
77. See Supplement VII.
78. *The Mahatma Letters to A.P. Sinnett. From the Mahatmas M. and K.H.*, third and revised edition 1979, Adyar, India. Letter no. 6.

79. See further regarding the two aspects of the Sun in: Sergei O. Prokofieff, *The Twelve Holy Nights and the Spiritual Hierarchies*, second edition, Temple Lodge Publishing 1993.
80. Op. cit., from letter no. 22. The quotation that follows is from letter no. 9.
81. Op. cit., from letter no. 23b.
82. See further regarding Christ's descent to the Earth through the cosmic spheres in: Sergei O. Prokofieff, *The Twelve Holy Nights and the Spiritual Hierarchies*, op. cit.
83. GA 211, lecture of 24 April 1922.
84. GA 116, lecture of 25 October 1909. See also the lectures in GA 113, 114 and 130.
85. GA 227, lecture of 29 August 1923.
86. GA 137, lecture of 12 June 1912.
87. GA 243, lecture of 20 August 1924.
88. GA 132, lecture of 31 October 1911.
89. Op. cit., from letter no. 22.
90. GA 136, lecture of 13 April 1912.
91. See Supplement VII.
92. GA 15, chapter III. See further in GA 114.
93. See Supplement VII.
94. GA 107, lecture of 22 March 1909.
95. See GA 113, lecture of 31 August 1909 and GA 264, the esoteric lesson of 1 June 1907.
96. GA 143, lecture of 8 May 1912.
97. GA 133, lecture of 23 October 1911.
98. *HR I*, 8 September 1934.
99. *HR I*, 15 November 1934.
100. *HR II*, 22 June 1936.
101. *HR II*, 24 May 1936 and *AY*.
102. *HR II*, 13 August 1938.
103. *HR II*, 24 September 1935.
104. *HR II*, 31 July 1937.
105. GA 137, lecture of 12 June 1912.
106. GA 133, lecture of 20 June 1912.
107. GA 131, lecture of 14 October 1911.
108. GA 28.
109. GA 143, lecture of 8 May 1912.

110. *AY.*
111. *PB.*
112. See note 33.
113. *HR II*, 23 July 1936.
114. *HR II*, 7 December 1935.
115. *HR I*, 6 May 1934.
116. *HR I*, 25 March 1935.
117. Ibid.
118. Ibid. and *HR II*, 30 March 1936.
119. *HR II*, 7 December 1935.
120. *HR I*, 21 July 1934.
121. *HR I*, 8 September 1934.
122. GA 116, lecture of 8 May 1910.
123. Ibid.
124. GA 130, lecture of 27 September 1911.
125. GA 143, lecture of 8 May 1912.
126. *AY.*
127. Ibid.
128. *HR I*, 24 June 1935.
129. Ibid.
130. See *Heart of Asia*, Roerich Museum Press, New York 1930.
131. See note 33.
132. GA 254, lecture of 17 October 1915.
133. Ibid.
134. *HR II*, 7 December 1935.
135. *HR I*, 20 April 1935.
136. *AY.*
137. *HR I*, 8 August 1934.
138. *HR I*, 12 April 1935.
139. *HR II*, 4 November 1935.
140. GA 131, lecture of 14 October 1911.
141. See GA 130, lecture of 4 November 1911 and other lectures in the same volume.
142. See GA 118.
143. GA 118, lecture of 10 May 1910.
144. GA 130, lecture of 21 September 1911.
145. GA 123, lecture of 10 September 1910.
146. GA 118, lecture of 6 March 1910.

147. *HR II*, 30 August 1935.
148. GA 130.
149. *HR II*, 30 March 1936.
150. GA 171.
151. Ibid.
152. See note 33.
153. *HR II*, 2 April 1936.
154. *HR II*, 30 March 1936.
155. *HR II*, 2 April 1936.
156. *AY*.
157. GA 109/111, lecture of 11 April 1909.
158. Ibid.
159. Ibid.
160. See GA 112, lecture of 6 July 1909.
161. See the lecture of 1 October 1911 (GA 130), 'The Etherisation of the Blood. The Entry of the Etheric Christ into Earthly Evolution'.
162. Ibid.
163. *HR I*, 30 April 1935.
164. GA 130, lecture of 18 December 1912.
165. *HR I*, 21 May 1935.
166. See GA 118.
167. *HR II*, 23 April 1938.
168. *HR II*, 1 October 1935 and 24 May 1936.
169. See GA 177.
170. *HR II*, 31 July 1937.
171. GA 254, lecture of 18 October 1915.

Notes to the Appendix

1. *Znamya mira. Gazyeta dukhovnovo yedinyeniya*, no. 7–8 (9–10) for the year 1993, p. 10, article by V. Kleshchevsky.
2. *LMG*.
3. V. Sidorov writes in connection with this in his postscript to the book *Zhivaya etica. Izbrannoye* ('Living Ethics. Selections'), Moscow 1992 (consisting of selected sections from the 14 volumes of Helena Roerich's *Agni Yoga*): 'It is to the highest degree curious and, of course, significant that in virtually all Western publications of the books of Living Ethics [Agni Yoga]

the theme of Russia is muffled and obscured. The first sentence of the first book is in such cases either omitted or edited and then given the following form: "To the New Country – My first proclamation".'

4. *FM.*
5. V. Sidorov writes about this: 'So the Roerichs did not consider themselves to be the authors of the books of 'Living Ethics' (*Agni Yoga*), as they asserted on more than one occasion . . . The Roerichs considered that their role was that of a connecting link between the mahatmas and humanity, that they were channels and transmitters for the teaching of the mahatmas' (see note 3).
6. The complete edition of all 14 books of *Agni Yoga* in three volumes, Vol. I, Samara 1992, book 4 *Znaki Agni yogi* ('Signs of Agni Yoga').
7. *COM.*
8. Helena Roerich, *Osnovy Buddizma* ('The Foundations of Buddhism'), a publication of the Siberian Roerich Society, Novosibirsk 1991.
9. Publisher's foreword to *COM* [Russian edition].
10. Quoted from *PB.*
11. N. Roerich, *Altai-Himalaya*, entry of 23 April 1926, Moscow, 1974. In publishing these diary entries from Roerich's great Himalayan expedition, the Soviet censor omitted from E. Chin-Ben's words the names of the founders of Buddhism and Christianity and replaced them with ellipses – probably because he reckoned the comparison to be inappropriate (after all, Lenin was a convinced materialist). However, in 1993, in the post-Bolshevik era, they could be published in full, without cuts, and were even included as the epigraph to an article on the relationship of the Roerichs to Lenin and to Bolshevism. See note 1.
12. V. Sidorov, foreword to *COM* [Russian edition].
13. Regarding the *Western* occult sources of Bolshevism, see note 37.
14. GA 181, lecture of 9 July 1918.
15. GA 181, lecture of 30 July 1918.
16. GA 192, lecture of 13 July 1919.

17. GA 192, lecture of 3 August 1919.
18. GA 198, lecture of 3 April 1920.
19. GA 293, lecture of 25 August 1919.
20. GA 192, lecture of 29 June 1919.
21. GA 197, lecture of 13 June 1920. The next quotation is from the same source.
22. Regarding the deeper occult foundations of Bolshevism, see the book referred to in note 37.
23. GA 294, lecture of 22 August 1919.
24. GA 198, lecture of 3 April 1920.
25. GA 182, lecture of 30 April 1918.
26. GA 199, lecture of 7 August 1920.

List of Works by Rudolf Steiner referred to in the Present Book

The English title is given only in cases where a comparable volume to the original German edition from the collected works – the *Gesamtausgabe* (abbreviated as 'GA') – has been published in English translation. In many cases, lectures are available in typescript or in print as single lectures or compilations from the collected works. For information on these contact Rudolf Steiner House Library, 35 Park Road, London NW1 6XT, or similar anthroposophical libraries around the world.

Publishers:

AP:	Anthroposophic Press (New York)
APC:	Anthroposophical Publishing Company (London)
GAR:	Garber Communications, Inc. (New York). Imprint: Spiritual Science Library
MER:	Mercury Press (Spring Valley, New York)
RSP:	Rudolf Steiner Press (Bristol)

Writings:

GA 11	*Cosmic Memory* (1904–08, GAR 1990)
GA 13	*Occult Science* (1910, RSP 1962)
GA 15	*The Spiritual Guidance of the Individual and Humanity* (1911, AP 1992)
GA 26	*Anthroposophical Leading Thoughts. Anthroposophy as a Path of Knowledge. The Michael Mystery* (1924–25, RSP 1985)
GA 28	*The Course of My Life* (1923–25, AP 1980)

Lectures:

GA 62	*Ergebnisse der Geistesforschung* (14 lectures, Berlin 1912–13)
GA 107	*Geisteswissenschaftliche Menschenkunde* (19 lectures, Berlin 1908–9)

GA 109/111 *Das Prinzip der spirituellen Ökonomie im Zusammenhang mit Wiederverkörperungsfragen. Ein Aspekt der geistigen Führung der Menschheit* (23 lectures given in various towns, 1909). Some lectures appear in *The Principle of Spiritual Economy* (AP 1986)

GA 110 *The Spiritual Hierarchies and their Reflection in the Physical World. Zodiac, Planets, Cosmos* (10 lectures, Düsseldorf 1909, AP 1983)

GA 112 *The Gospel of St John and its Relation to the Other Gospels, especially to that of St Luke* (14 lectures, Kassel 1909, AP 1982)

GA 113 *The East in the Light of the West. The Children of Lucifer and the Brothers of Christ* (9 lectures, Munich 1909, GAR 1986)

GA 114 *The Gospel of St Luke* (10 lectures, Basel 1909, RSP 1988)

GA 116 *The Christ Impulse and the Development of Ego Consciousness* (7 lectures, Berlin 1909–10, AP 1976)

GA 118 *Das Ereignis der Christus-Erscheinung in der ätherischen Welt* (16 lectures given in various towns, 1909). Some lectures appear in *The Reappearance of Christ in the Etheric* (AP 1985)

GA 123 *The Gospel of St Matthew* (12 lectures, Bern 1910, RSP 1985)

GA 129 *Wonders of the World, Ordeals of the Soul, Revelations of the Spirit* (11 lectures, Munich 1911, RSP 1983)

GA 130 *Das esoterische Christentum und die geistige Führung der Menschheit* (23 lectures given in various towns, 1911–12)

GA 131 *From Jesus to Christ* (11 lectures, Karlsruhe 1911, RSP 1991)

GA 132 *The Inner Realities of Evolution* (5 lectures, Berlin 1911, RSP 1953)

GA 133 *Earthly and Cosmic Man* (9 lectures, Berlin 1911–12)

GA 136 *The Spiritual Beings in the Heavenly Bodies and in the Kingdoms of Nature* (11 lectures, Helsinki 1912, GAR 1986)

GA 137 *Man in the Light of Occultism, Theosophy and Philosophy* (10 lectures, Christiana, Oslo, 1912, GAR 1989)

GA 143	*Erfahrungen des Übersinnlichen. Die Wege der Seele zu Christus* (14 lectures given in various towns, 1912)
GA 145	*The Effect of Spiritual Development* (10 lectures, The Hague 1913, RSP 1978)
GA 158	*Der Zusammenhang des Menschen mit der elementarischen Welt. Kalewala, Olaf Åsteson. Das russische Volkstum. Die Welt als Ergebnis von Gleichgewichtswirkungen* (10 lectures given in various towns, 1912–14)
GA 167	*Gegenwärtiges und Vergangenes im Menschengeiste* (12 lectures, Berlin 1916)
GA 171	*Inner impulses of Evolution* (16 lectures, Dornach 1916, AP 1984)
GA 172	*The Karma of Vocation* (10 lectures, Dornach 1916, AP 1984)
GA 174a	*Kosmische und Menschliche Geschichte VI: Mitteleuropa zwischen Ost und West* (12 lectures, Munich 1914–18)
GA 177	*The Fall of the Spirits of Darkness* (14 lectures, Dornach 1918, RSP 1993)
GA 181	*Earthly Death and Cosmic Life* (21 lectures, Berlin 1918, GAR 1989)
GA 182	*Der Tod als Lebenswandlung* (7 lectures given in various towns, 1917–18)
GA 191	*Die geistigen Hintergründe der sozialen Frage III: Soziales Verständnis aus geisteswissenschaftlicher Erkenntnis* (15 lectures, Dornach 1919)
GA 192	*Geisteswissenschaftliche Behandlung sozialer und pädagogischen Fragen* (17 lectures, Stuttgart 1919)
GA 193	*Der innere Aspekt des sozialen Rätsels. Luziferische Vergangenheit und ahrimanische Zukunft* (10 lectures given in various towns, 1919). Some lectures appear in *The Inner Aspect of the Social Question* (RSP 1974)
GA 194	*Die Sendung Michaels. Die Offenbarung der eigentlichen Geheimnisse des Menschenwesens* (12 lectures, Dornach 1919). Some lectures appear in *The Mission of the Archangel Michael* (AP 1961)
GA 195	*The Cosmic New Year* (5 lectures, Stuttgart 1919–20)
GA 196	*Geistige und soziale Wandlungen in der Menschheitsentwicklung* (18 lectures, Dornach 1920, APC 1932)

GA 197 *Polarities in the Evolution of Mankind* (11 lectures, Stuttgart 1920, RSP 1987)

GA 198 *Heilfaktoren für den sozialen Organismus* (17 lectures, Dornach and Bern 1920)

GA 199 *Spiritual Science as a Foundation for Social Forms* (17 lectures, Dornach and Berlin 1920, AP 1986)

GA 201 *Man – Hieroglyph of the Universe* (16 lectures, Dornach 1920, RSP 1972)

GA 202 *Der Mensch in seinem Zusammenhang mit dem Kosmos II. Die Brücke zwischen der Weltgeistigkeit und dem Physischen des Menschen. Die Suche nach der neuen Isis, der göttlichen Sophia* (16 lectures, Dornach, Bern and Basel, 1920)

GA 211 *Das Sonnenmysterium und das Mysterium von Tod und Auferstehung. Exoterisches und esoterisches Christentum* (12 lectures given in various towns, 1922)

GA 227 *The Evolution of Consciousness* (13 lectures, Penmaenmawr 1923, RSP 1966)

GA 243 *True and False Paths in Spiritual Investigation* (11 lectures, Torquay 1924, RSP 1985)

GA 254 *The Occult Movement in the Nineteenth Century* (13 lectures, Dornach 1915, RSP 1973)

GA 258 *The Anthroposophic Movement* (8 lectures, Dornach 1923, RSP 1993)

GA 262 *Correspondence and Documents, Rudolf Steiner and Marie Steiner-von Sivers* (1901–25, RSP 1988)

GA 264 *Zur Geschichte und aus den Inhalten der ersten Abteilung der Esoterischen Schule von 1904 bis 1914*

GA 293 *Study of Man* (14 lectures, Stuttgart 1919, RSP 1990)

GA 294 *Practical Advice to Teachers* (14 lectures, Stuttgart 1919, RSP 1988)

By the same author:

The Cycle of the Year as a Path of Initiation
Eternal Individuality, Towards a Karmic Biography of Novalis
The Occult Significance of Forgiveness
Prophecy of the Russian Epic
Rudolf Steiner and the Founding of the New Mysteries
The Spiritual Origins of Eastern Europe and the Future Mysteries of the Holy Grail
The Twelve Holy Nights and the Spiritual Hierarchies

For a free catalogue write to:
Temple Lodge Publishing
51 Queen Caroline Street
London W6 9QL